AF527982

Anthropology and Health Issues

Anthropology and Health Issues

Edited by

Buddhadeb Chaudhuri
Subir Biswas

Indira Gandhi Rashtriya Manav Sangrahalaya, Bhopal
(National Museum of Mankind)

RAWAT PUBLICATIONS
Jaipur • New Delhi • Bangalore • Hyderabad • Guwahati • Kolkata

ISBN 978-81-316-0669-8

© Indira Gandhi Rashtriya Manav Sangrahalaya, Bhopal, 2014

No part of this book may be reproduced or transmitted in any form or by any means, electronic or mechanical, including photocopying, recording or by any information storage and retrieval system, without permission in writing from the publishers.

The responsibility for the facts stated, opinions expressed or conclusions reached, are entirely that of the authors and that IGRMS, Bhopal accepts no responsibility for them.

Published by
Indira Gandhi Rashtriya Manav Sangrahalaya
Shamla Hills, Bhopal-462013 (Madhya Pradesh)
email: directorigrms@gmail.com

Prem Rawat for **Rawat Publications**
Satyam Apts, Sector 3, Jawahar Nagar, Jaipur 302 004 (India)
Phone: 0141 265 1748 / 7006 Fax: 0141 265 1748
E-mail: info@rawatbooks.com
Website: www.rawatbooks.com

New Delhi Office
4858/24, Ansari Road, Daryaganj, New Delhi 110 002
Phone: 011 2326 3290

Also at *Bangalore, Hyderabad, Guwahati* and *Kolkata*

Typeset by Rawat Computers, Jaipur
Printed at Chaman Enterprises, New Delhi

Contents

Preface

An International Conference on 'Mega-Urbanisation and Human Rights: Emerging Challenges and Opportunities' was organised in Kolkata (Calcutta) during 14–16 February 2011. It was jointly organised by Commission on Urban Anthropology, Commission on Human Rights of International Union of Anthropological and Ethnological Sciences and the Department of Anthropology, West Bengal State University and sponsored by Indira Gandhi Rashtriya Manav Sangrahalaya, Anthropological Survey of India, Indian Council of Social Science Research, Indian Council of Medical Research and Indian Museum and Centre for Alternative Research in Development. We received 124 papers from Bangladesh, Chile, Mexico, USA, Canada, Greece, Turkey, UK, Nepal and different parts of India. These papers were presented in 20 sessions, organised on different aspects of urbanisation and human rights. The issue of health was discussed in a number of sessions covering various health aspects in the context of urbanisation and human rights. The present volume includes 15 articles exclusively dealing with health, presented in different sessions of this international conference.

II

Medical practitioners and public health workers often report that people do not utilise the medical and preventive facilities available to them. The interacting influences of socio-cultural milieu towards the essentially biological and physical maladies needs deep analyses. Social and economic factors are generally accepted as highly important in the multiple causation of disease. Therefore, health workers must come to understand such factors if they are to deal effectively in both primary prevention and cure of disease and other disorders of health. Another important factor is socio-psychological. When a person goes to a traditional medicine man, one gets something more beyond physical health. It is the socio-psychological reinforcement, which one cannot get from the western medical practitioner. Anthropological studies covering different facets of the society are urgently necessary to understand some of the realities of health problems. The environment, sanitation, habits of the people, food and level of nutrition are other important aspects which need to be considered. Besides these, knowledge and documentation of traditional medicine are also urgently necessary. A study of indigenous methods of treatment may help to identify new methods of treatment of various diseases with certain modifications. In fact, in many parts of the world, a number of ethno-botanical studies have helped to identify a number of medicinal plants to treat different types of diseases. It is urgently necessary to document them and try them after proper scientific experiment.

In the context of present globalisation process and Patent Acts, the knowledge system and herbal medicines have a very different significance and implications. The resources, particularly in the developing countries, are very limited. In this context, it is to be seen how best we can utilise the resources and the health policies are to be critically examined. Should we go for more expensive sophisticated health facilities serving only a few or minimum health facilities to a large population? What should be the priority? Again, in the contemporary world, one cannot deny the various hazards connected with different jobs. These are the emerging health challenges based on changing socio-cultural and economic situation. One will have to address and examine some of these new health problems. Many of these issues have been examined in the present volume.

III

There are three sections in the present volume. Section I on 'Health Issues and Human Rights' has five chapters. Section II on 'Occupation and Health: The Challenges' has four chapters. The last section on 'Changing Health Scenario: Opportunities and Challenges' comprises six chapters.

In chapter one, Nita Mawar point at bio-ethics scholars who have identified human rights and social justice as key considerations for biomedical and health research. The potential for addressing human rights considerations in international health research has been proven through approaches that include collaborative partnerships, capacity building, and respect for cultural traditions. She stresses that there is a growing need to understand the relation and inter-sections between health research, ethics and human rights. This need becomes even more imperative in the era of globalisation and mega-urbanisation, especially when global health research through international funding is on the rise. She further suggests that to address the complexities, building capacities at local communities is required. Further, a commitment to an engaged dialogue and action among investigators, funding agencies, policy makers, governmental institutions, and private industry is crucial. Overall, there is a need to create an ambience that enhances the much needed skill and capacity for critical and informed reflection that transcends from health research ethics to the rights of the local community.

The main issue taken up by Sonia Chacko and Bini Toms in chapter two is the role of Intellectual Property Rights (IPRs) and IPRs' organisations in health research, with particular emphasis on the protection of rights of researchers. The existing number of organisations dealing with IPRs has been examined and its increase in recent years has been reviewed. An effort has been made to study the number of IPR organisations dealing exclusively with health research IPRs. Finally, note has been taken that with increasing urbanisation, as collaboration between researchers, both local and international, continue to increase, the rights of the less influential researchers, be it local or international can be protected through IPRs.

In chapter three, S.K. Nandy and others examine the issue of mental health and make a critical review of this emerging health problem in urban areas and often resulting due to various social strains.

Bini Toms, in chapter four, has pointed out that industrialisation and improved agricultural practices are resulting in growing genetic erosion of plant resources. Today, there are just 150 crops which feed the people on this planet as compared to 10,000 plant species at the dawn of agriculture. Loss of biodiversity is one of the seven indicators of unacceptable environmental changes and therefore, conservation of plant genetic diversity would be one of the most effective ways to prevent these unacceptable changes. The issue of plant genetic diversity conservation is very important because it is one of the most effective ways to prevent climatic changes and ensure human sustenance. She stresses that the combined efforts of plant scientists, government and the general public as a whole in this direction is the need of the hour to arrest this irreversible loss of plant genetic biodiversity.

In chapter five, Pranjal Boruah examines the health and educational rights of the children in an urban slum. As the parents are uneducated, they do not encourage their children for education. This results in their children being deprived of right to education.

The government educational scheme like *Sarva Sikhsa Abhiyan* do not reach these areas. The paper also includes a few suggestions on the future strategy for their entire improvement.

In chapter six, Guddi Tiwary and P.K. Gangopadhyay note that construction is one of the important industries employing large number of workforce. A wide range of activities are involved in it. Due to advent of industrialisation and recent developments, this industry is taking a pivotal role for construction of buildings, roads, bridges etc. The workers engaged in this industry, are victims of different occupational disorders and psychosocial stresses. An attempt has also been made to review some of the available important articles for highlighting the problem faced by this working group.

Sovan Chakraborty, in chapter seven, discusses about cycle rickshaw wallas, one of the most important category of the informal sector in the urban setting. The growing informal sectors in the mega cities in India have provided economic opportunities to the immigrant population. Owing to disparity in economic development among different regions, people from one region migrate to the other, towards the metropolitan centre. This chapter focuses on socio-economic condition and the health of the cycle rickshaw wallas of Kolkata.

Jokhan Sharma and others have examined and explored the health and socio-economic status of rag-picker children with special reference to Hazaribagh region. The work exposes the health hazards and different kind of problems, which affect their overall future development.

In chapter nine, Swapna Vijayan and others examine the health problem of urban women executives. They noted that the persistent stress induced by the craze to attain goals has a chronic underlying effect which adversely affects the physiological homeostasis of executives, making them prone to metabolic disorders and diseases. Besides, irregular and undesirable food habits are contributory to this urbanisation induced lifestyle disorder.

Parama Ukil, in chapter ten, examines the effects of urbanisation and globalisation on women's health. She notes that several declarations and targets are available for improving the condition of women's health. But there is question regarding their implementation. This chapter also specifically examined the Millennium Development Goals regarding poor/marginalised women's health and how far the targets have been achieved. Whether the goals are sufficient to protect and ensure women's right to health have also been noted.

In chapter eleven, Rimi Dutta and Pinak Tarafdar discuss the health situation and health care issues of the Totos of North Bengal, one of the primitive tribal groups in West Bengal.

In chapter twelve, Shruti Agrawal and Pratiti Ghosh discuss the health of scheduled caste women in West Bengal and Bihar. It has been noted that the backward castes of both the states in the urban suburbs or in the town are found to be over-burdened and are devoid of minimum amenities like quality drinking water or kitchen or even electricity. This study reveals that mega-urbanisation has insignificantly elevated the health-style of the scheduled castes residing in the suburbs of the cities and mega cities.

Basavanagouda T.T., in chapter thirteen, discusses the health seeking behaviour of Kudubi community of South Kanara, Karnataka. In order to understand health and hygiene of this community, house types, sanitary habits, food habits, work and leisure practices and the level of their understanding of the concept of health and hygiene is covered. It was found that, Kudubi rarely seek the help of modern medicine for minor complaints like cough, cold and common fever etc. For these ailments, remedies are given in the home by elderly persons who possess rich experience in life. In case of major complaints, they seek the help from the doctors of primary health centre in the village or private doctors.

In chapter fourteen, D.K. Adak and N.K. Bagchi note about the problem of cardiovascular disease which is growing in magnitude in the developing countries like India. Though there are a good number of epidemiological studies on cardiovascular disease in India, such type of study are scanty in Central India. Present study is an endeavour to deal with epidemiology of cardiovascular disease in an urban centre of Central India, namely Sagar town of Madhya Pradesh. The study reveals that variables like hypertension, family history of cardiac disorder, level of education and obesity showed significant relationship with cardiovascular disease.

In the last chapter, V. Jagadeesh studies the changing health seeking behaviour of the Banjaras of Karnataka. He notes that traditional societies like Banjaras are well adapted to their environments and that their members are healthy and nourished. But a change in the environment has affected the situation and is adversely affecting the health.

IV

The editors record with appreciation, the support received from Indira Gandhi Rashtriya Manav Sangrahalaya, Anthropological Survey of India, Indian Council of Social Science Research, Indian Council of Medical Research, Indian Museum and Centre for Alternative Research in Development. It was possible to organise the conference successfully only through the active support of students and faculty members of Department of Anthropology, West Bengal State University and members of Centre for Alternative Research in Development. We are grateful to Professor Ashoke Ranjan Thakur, the then Honourable Vice-Chancellor of the University, for his keen interest, kind guidance, financial support, as well as active participation. He not only chaired the inaugural session, but also participated in a few other sessions. We are also grateful to Professor Asis Kumar Banerjee, former Vice-Chancellor, Calcutta University for delivering the valedictory address and his keen interest and kind guidance. We are thankful to all the delegates from various parts of the world for their active participation. Special thanks are due to Dr Sumia Chaudhuri, Co-Convener of the conference for her valuable help and contribution to organise the conference as well as for publication of the first volume (present volume is one of the several volumes to be edited by organisers and mostly concentrated on human health issues, specially impact of urbanisation on human health). Special thanks to Director, Indira Gandhi Rashtriya Manav Sangrahalaya for his interest and initiative for publication.

Buddhadeb Chaudhuri
Subir Biswas

Contributors

D.K. Adak, Research Associate (P), Anthropological Survey of India, 27, Jawaharlal Nehru Road, Kolkata.
Email: adakdipak@gmail.com

Shruti Agrawal, Lecturer, Department of Food and Nutrition, GMSM Mahavidyalaya, Bireswarpur, South 24 Parganas, West Bengal.
Email: shrutiagrawal74@yahoo.co.in

N.K. Bagchi, Research Associate (P), Anthropological Survey of India, 27, Jawaharlal Nehru Road, Kolkata.
Email: niloy.bagchi@rediffmail.com

Pranjal Boruah, Assistant Professor, Department of Anthropology, Dibru College, Dibrugarh.
Email: anthroboruah@yahoo.co.in

Sonia Chacko, Faculty, Department of Biosciences, T. John College, Bangalore.
Email: soniachacko@rediffmail.com

Sovan Chakraborty, ICSSR Doctoral Fellow, Department of Anthropology, University of Calcutta, 35, Ballygunge Circular Road, Kolkata.
Email: chakraborty.sovan@gmail.com

Suniti Chatterjee, Associate Professor, Department of Home Science, University of Calcutta, 20B, Judges Court Road, Alipore, Kolkata.
Email: sunitighoshchatterji@gmail.com.

Abhishek Chauhan, Research Scholar, Department of Anthropology, Ranchi University, Ranchi, Jharkhand.
Email: chauhan1984@rediffmail.com.

Supurna Das, Consultant Psychologist, Mind Care Clinic, P–256, Block B, Lake Town, Kolkata.

Rimi Dutta, Research Scholar, Department of Anthropology, North Bengal University, Raja Rammohanpur, Darjeeling, West Bengal.
Email: rimi_nbu@rediffmail.com

P.K. Gangopadhyay, Scientist-F, Regional Occupational Health Centre (E), (Indian Council of Medical Research), Block DP–1, Salt Lake City, Kolkata.
Email: gangulipk@yahoo.co.in

Pratiti Ghosh, Associate Professor and Head, Department of Physiology, West Bengal State University, Kolkata.
Email: pratiti_ghosh@yahoo.co.in

V. Jagadeesh, Associate Professor, Department of Anthropology, Karnatak College of Karnatak University, Dharwad.
Email: drvjagadeesh@gmail.com

Alok Kumar, Research Scholar, Department of Anthropology, Vinobha Bhave University, Hazaribagh, Jharkhand.
Email: alokanthrovbu77@gmail.com

Nita Mawar, Scientist 'F'/Deputy Director-Senior Grade and HOD, Social and Behavioural Research Division, National AIDS Research Institute (ICMR), 73–G, Bhosari Industrial Estate, Pune.
Email: nmawar@nariindia.org and nmawar2@gmail.com

Amitava Mukherji, Consultant Psychiatrist, Mind Care Clinic, P–256, Block B, Lake Town, Kolkata.
Email: dramitera@vsnl.net

Shyamal Kumar Nandy, Research Associate (C), Anthropological Survey of India (ERC), EN–79 Sector–V, Salt Lake, Kolkata.
Email: shymlnandy@yahoo.com

Jokhan Sharma, Project Research Assistant at Anthropological Survey of India, North-West Regional Centre, 192/1, Kaulagarh Road, Dehradun.
Email: jokhansharma@gmail.com

Basavanagouda T.T., Associate Professor, P.G. Department of Anthropology, Karnatak University, Dharwad.
Email: drbasavanagoudatt@gmail.com

Pinak Tarafdar, Assistant Professor, Department of Anthropology, North Bengal University, Raja Rammohunpur, Darjeeling, West Bengal.
Email: pinak_anth@rediffmail.com

Guddi Tiwary, Senior Research Fellow, Regional Occupational Health Centre (E), Block – DP, No. 1; Salt Lake City, Kolkata.
Email: guddi190@gmail.com

Bini Toms, Fogarty Fellow, Joint Centre for Bioethics, University of Toronto, Canada.
Email: bini_toms@yahoo.co.in

Parama Ukil, UGC Senior Research Fellow, Women's Studies Research Centre, University of Calcutta, Alipore Campus. 1, Reformatory Street, Kolkata.
Email: parama.ukil@gmail.com

Swapna Vijayan, Lecturer, Department of Food and Nutrition, Acharya Prafulla Chandra College, New Barrackpore, Kolkata.
Email: samirmukherjee@gmail.com

SECTION I

Health Issues and Human Rights

CHAPTER 1

Reviewing Health Research, Ethics and Human Rights

Where and How Do They Connect?

NITA MAWAR

Recognising the impact of structural issues on global health including socio-economic and political factors, bio-ethics scholars have identified human rights and social justice as key considerations for biomedical and health research. The potential for addressing human rights considerations in international health research has been proven through approaches that include collaborative partnerships, capacity building, and respect for cultural traditions.

This works on a framework that is the basis of the ethical principle of respect for autonomy and maintaining confidentiality, beneficence and no harm done to the subject(s) and non-discriminatory procedures that eliminate bias against choosing a specific group who may not stand to gain from this research. This includes bio-medical intervention, social intervention; this also includes testing of a product made in a developing country to be tried in a developing country, covering communities who may not benefit from such product/intervention in the near future (ICMR, 2006).

Issue

There is a growing need to understand the relation and inter-sections between health research, ethics and human rights in a better way. This need becomes even more imperative in the era of globalisation and mega-urbanisation, especially when global health research through international funding is on the rise.

Medical ethics: A system of moral principles that apply values and judgements to the practice of medicine. As a scholarly discipline, medical ethics encompasses its practical application in clinical settings as well as work on its history, philosophy, theology, and sociology (ICMR, 2006; IILP, 2012; Marshal, 2005; NCESSRH, 2000).

Ethical issues in research essentially takes two forms: the structural (economic and political) and the particular or relational, both of which deserve attention. The second form is understood as the kinds of interactions that take place between researchers and participants and those matters that are the traditional focus of ethical review. Since research ethics adopts a clinical model, this focus seems natural.

Structural is understood in terms of where the power rests and who makes decisions about what research is to be done, why should it be done, in whose interests and what and who gets left behind. Far more ethical energy is directed towards the personal, possibly because it seems manageable. Even so, our systems for scrutinising research practice have marginal impact on the ways in which research might be conducted. A great deal depends upon how researchers interpret their responsibilities and the intentions of the funders of research.

Human rights are 'rights and freedoms to which all humans are entitled'. Proponents of the concept usually assert that everyone is endowed with certain entitlements merely by reason of being human. Human rights are thus conceived in a Universalist and egalitarian fashion. Such entitlements can exist as shared norms of actual human moralities, as justified moral norms or natural rights supported by strong reasons, or as legal rights either at a national level or within international law (Loff, 2011; Marshall, 2005).

However, there is no consensus as to the precise nature of what in particular should or should not be regarded as a human right in any of the preceding senses, and the abstract concept of human rights has been a subject of intense philosophical debate and criticism.

Many of the basic ideas that animated the movement developed in the aftermath of the Second World War, culminating in its adoption by the Universal Declaration of Human Rights by the United Nations General Assembly in 1948. The true forerunner of human rights discourse was the enlightenment concept of natural rights developed by figures such as John Locke and Immanuel Kant and through the political realm in the United States Bill of Rights and the Declaration of the Rights of Man and of the Citizen (Loff, 2011; Marshall, 2005; Nickel, 2007, 2009; UN General assembly, 1948).

> All human beings are born free and equal in dignity and rights. They are endowed with reason and conscience and should act towards one another in a spirit of brotherhood. (UN, 1948)
>
> — Article 1 of the United Nations Universal Declaration of Human Rights (UDHR, UNGA, 1948)

Importance of Ethics in Health Research

Society has an intrinsic interest in ensuring that all human activity is conducted sensitively, in the interest of others, and after a process of informed understanding, i.e., through comprehension and reflection. This is where enhancing capacity building programmes among researchers through strengthening professional knowledge on research ethics becomes pertinent. This includes increasing awareness of ethical concerns associated with varied study designs and informed consent processes among researchers.

In addition, technological and financial resources are necessary to build capacity at the level of local communities to enable the integration of research results into existing health systems. This should be possible through the application of ethical guidelines within the cultural context of the community to address the human rights (ICMR, 2006; Loff, 2011; NCESSRH, 2000; Nickel, 2009).

Research with Vulnerable Populations

Research with vulnerable should be conducted very carefully and with respect. Vulnerability is understood as the deprivation of basic human rights and/or an inability to exercise those rights. The research in these populations is not likely to alter their situation of vulnerability (Loff, 2011; Marshall, 2005).

The likelihood is that the researcher/sponsor/funder is using the participant instrumentally (though not necessarily consciously or intentionally), and that, the researcher/sponsor/funder, may as a result of doing the research, prosper in some way. Even if the participant derives some sort of benefit, it may not be meaningful to them. The research process may ultimately be burdensome, having failed to produce any sustainable long-term or even short-term improvement of basic rights.

Research among the vulnerable groups need to be conducted with caution, keeping the dignity and respect of those who are covered within this group. Many of the researches done among these populations are unlikely to alter their vulnerabilities and are probably not intended to do so. One of the recent developments that brought up this pertinent aspect is the Universal Declaration on Bioethics and Human Rights from UNESCO, which addresses States, individuals, groups, communities, institutions and corporations, public and private. However, ethical obligations and the intersections with human rights that apply beyond the relationship of researcher with the participant still remains inadequately articulated.

Who is Responsible for Addressing these Ethical Requirements?

States, by virtue of their legislative, economic powers and human rights obligations are responsible for addressing ethical requirements. Multi and bilateral agencies, corporate bodies and others whether private or public are also part of it.

While the proportion of clinical research conducted in the developing world is rising, most clinical research is carried out in the United States by pharmaceutical companies. Having more confidence in the potential impact of regulatory mechanisms such as these ethical obligations than the less specific requirements contained in ethical guidelines is being recognised. However, at the same time the developing countries need to focus attention on educating their own population to be able to take on these responsibilities.

How Else Can Low and Middle Income Countries Safeguard Themselves against Exploitation in Research?

This requires a significant will on the part of government. Ultimately for reasons to redress the inherent exploitative nature of such research, the research content and process must also direct itself towards lessening the vulnerability of the population by attending to the improvement of their basic rights. This can only happen by ensuring consistency with a programme of development that is directed towards improvement of human well-being and not simply economic productivity.

The Needed Ethical Capacity for Researchers

It is important to reshape the way we think of ethics in research and make all research partners ethically accountable in different ways. This includes the research partners at varied levels: the sponsors and/or funding agency, the country, institution and the research team where it is carried out and the individual and community researched upon. Research ethics and our current system of ethical review primarily consider the relationship between the researcher and the participant – and on occasion the participant community.

This makes it an unnecessarily limited vision. It means that those who really drive what happens in research escape rigorous scrutiny. It is significant to introspect by going back and improve the skill needed for capacity strengthening for critical and informed reflection in our understanding (Loff, 2011).

Conclusion

To address the complexities of research ethics and vulnerable populations and their rights especially with international funding, building capacities at local level, i.e., researchers in developing countries to the communities being researched is required. The right to health also requires states to affirmatively provide health information both to individuals and to medical professionals. States are also obligated to provide women with accurate information so as to ensure that children and adolescents have appropriate care. They are obligated to ensure that health workers receive adequate training and adequate access to relevant and medically accurate health information and to regulate interference by third parties.

Further, a commitment to an engaged dialogue and action among investigators, funding agencies, policy makers, governmental institutions, and private industry is crucial. Overall, there is a need to create an ambience that enhances the much needed skill and capacity for critical and informed reflection that transcends from health research ethics to the rights of the local community.

Acknowledgements: I would like to thank the NIH-ICMR Bio-ethics training programme in 2007, Bangalore which helped me in continuing my interest in ethics.

References

Barendt, E. 1997. 'Privacy as a Constitutional Right and Value', in P. Birks (ed.), *Privacy and Loyalty*. Clarendon Press, Oxford.

Indian Council of Medical Research (ICMR). 2006. *Ethical Guidelines for Biomedical Research on Human Participants*. ICMR, New Delhi.

Institute for Information Law and Policy (IILP). 2012. *Access to Health Information under International Human Rights Law*. IILP in cooperation with the Justice Action Center and Healthcare Information for all by 2015. White paper series 11/12/01.

Loff, B. 2011. *Improving Human Rights for Better Ethics in Research*. Council on Health Research for Development (COHRED). <http://www.cohred.org/perspectives/improving-human-rights-for-better-ethics-in-research/>. 14 February 2011.

Marshall, P.A. 2005. 'Human Rights, Cultural Pluralism, and International Health Research'. *Theoretical Medicine and Bioethics*, 26 (6): 529–57.

National Committee for Ethics in Social Science Research in Health (NCESSRH). 2000. *Ethical Guidelines for Research in Social Sciences and Health*. Centre for Equity into Health and Allied Themes, Mumbai.

Nickel, J. 2007. *Making Sense of Human Rights* (2nd ed.). Blackwell, London.

——. 2009. 'Human Rights', in N. Edward (ed.), *The Stanford Encyclopedia of Philosophy*. <http://plato.stanford.edu/archives/spr2009/entries/rights-human/10022011>. 14 February 2011.

United Nations. 1948. *Universal Declaration of Human Rights* adopted by General Assembly Resolution 217 A (III) of 10 December 1948.

CHAPTER 2

Intellectual Property Right in Human Health Research and Its Implications

A Review

SONIA CHACKO AND BINI TOMS

Intellectual property (IP) is the term that describes the ideas, inventions, technologies, artworks, music and literature, that are intangible when first created, but become valuable in tangible form as products. Intellectual properties are the creations of the mind: inventions, literary and artistic works, and the symbols, names, and designs used in commerce. The rationale for the establishment of a legal framework on IP is that it is a signal to society that creative and inventive ideas will be rewarded. This chapter is an attempt to review the role of Intellectual Property Right (IPR) in public health and what needs to be done in context to the advancement of science and technology.

Nature of IPR

Intellectual property rights as a collective term includes the following independent IP rights which can be collectively used for protecting different aspects of an inventive work for multiple protection: Patents, Copyrights, Trademarks,

Registered (industrial) design, Protection of integrated circuit (IC) layout design, Geographical indications, and Protection of undisclosed information design. IPR are largely territorial rights except copyright, which is global in nature in the sense that it is immediately available in all the members of the Berne Convention. These rights are awarded by the State. They are monopoly rights implying that no one can use these rights without the consent of the right holder. It is important to know that these rights have to be renewed from time to time for keeping them in force except in case of copyright and trademarks.

Each product is amalgamation of many different areas of science and technologies. Intellectual property plays an important role in an increasingly broad range of areas, ranging from the internet to health care to nearly all aspects of science and technology, literature and the arts. Thus to promote informed discussion and awareness of the intellectual property, education in this field is important.

Intellectual Property and Economic Development

The establishment of the World Trade Organization (WTO) in 1994, with the new General Agreement on Tariffs and Trade (GATT, 1994) and the International Agreement on Trade Related Aspects of Intellectual Property Rights (TRIPS) has far reaching implications on global economy. GATT resulted in gradual opening of international markets. The agreement on TRIPs, introduced mandatory international standards for the protection of IPRs for the first time in history, especially in the area of patents. Developments following the establishment of WTO are characterised not only by the globalisation of markets, but also by globalisation of research and development. Thus the advent of globalisation coined the term 'knowledge economy'.

During the last 10 years, IPRs have gained numerous economic importances, the reason being the rapid progress of science and technology, especially communication and information technology and biotechnology, which led to the establishment of new knowledge based industries (Straus, 2004). Thus the conceptualisation of knowledge as intellectual capital and the management of knowledge are identified with creating competitive advantage in the knowledge economy (Flood et al., 2002; Prahalad, 1990). Intellectual capital (IC) is identified with those components of knowledge that can be created through human capital and whose value can be identified and extracted (Harrison and Sullivan, 2000; WIPO, 2004).

However, there is constant criticism that IP is considered a barrier to access to life-saving medicine and critical technologies. Intellectual property protection drags down developing economies by resulting in loss of jobs, driving up prices on goods due to monopoly created by IP reducing access to technology needed for development, requiring developing countries to administer and enforce IP rights and compelling companies to pay licenses or royalties on the products that they produce. IPR imposes unjustifiable burdens, unfairly extracts value from developing countries, and pays inadequate attention to the protection of traditional knowledge.

However, the other side remains contradictory. Human creativity is a vast national resource for any country. Intellectual property protection is the tool that protects these resources. A strong intellectual property regime reassures potential investors that their capital and their technologies will not fall prey to piracy and counterfeiting. IP would encourage participation in the growing global technology networks by release of powerful internal resources. It could stimulate acquisition and dissemination of new information. Also evidences indicate that Indian Patent Act 2005 has had no negative impact on India's pharma industry. Indeed the industry is growing robust; moreover prices of medicines in India are among the lowest in the world.

Implication of Intellectual Property in the Bio-economy of 2030

It is assumed that the agricultural and health field will see the greatest impact of the above mentioned changes in biotechnological intellectual property in respect of the Bio-economy of 2030. To address concerns of climate change and food security as well as the increasing convergence of agricultural and health biotechnologies, pressure will increase on finding collaborative mechanisms to manage intellectual property. Hence simplified and standard Material Transfer Agreements and intellectual property license agreements will be required to sustain such collaborative research effort.

To obtain the full benefits of the Bio-economy in 2030 in health biotechnology, greater collaboration will be needed on at least two fronts. First, in order to overcome the increasing difficulty of identifying new drug targets, greater collaboration between industry partners and the public sector will be required. Second, to better enable regulators to evaluate the safety and efficacy of new medication, industry will need to share platforms with regulators across the world. Both sets of collaborations will depend on developing strategies that open access to proprietary technologies and to share the benefits arising from their use (Richard and Matthew, 2007).

Current Intellectual Property Management Issues in India

With the opening up of trade in goods and services intellectual property rights (IPR) have become more susceptible to infringement leading to inadequate return to the creators of knowledge. It is evident that in a developed economy a defined and long term commitment to Research and Development (R&D) is mandatory for sustained competitiveness. An R&D based economy needs a favourable environment. Government needs to implement several policies that encourage public and private sector R&D investment of direct benefit to the people of India. R&D is risky, expensive and has uncertain outcomes, hence the government needs to provide specific protection that create environment for focused research. The cost of introducing a new drug into the market may cost a company anywhere between $300 million to $600 million alongwith all the associated risks at the developmental stage. No company will like to risk its intellectual property becoming a public property without adequate returns. The lack of return in the absence of robust IPR protection will discourage further R&D and foreign investments.

The transition of India from a protected economy to be an open, global-economic power has prompted India to take a series of steps to face the new challenges of globalisation. Earlier experiences have shown that only through indigenous development, new health products could be developed, introduced and marketed. Strengthening R&D and establishing policies for the creation and management of IP and public-partnerships are important steps for making available products of public health importance in all poor countries. The pharmaceutical and biotechnology industries have been among the first to understand the implications of the new patent regime and the need to carry out innovative R&D. Even public sector institutions have realised the need to reconsider their IP policies. Agencies like the Indian Council of Medical Research (ICMR), Department of Biotechnology (DBT) has adopted IP policies to promote innovative R&D, encourage partnerships with industry, create incentives for patent filing and systems of royalty sharing with inventors, and so on.

Thus it is rightly said that knowledge and information, economically exploited as intellectual property are replacing the more traditional, material elements of production as the primary engine of economic growth. It is influenced by the ingenuity, creativity and innovative ability of a nation. Converting these resources into tangible economic assets requires an effective and efficient intellectual property system. Creating, obtaining, protecting, and managing intellectual property must become a corporate activity in the same manner as the raising of resources and funds. The knowledge revolution will demand a special pedestal for intellectual property in the overall decision making process (Saha, 2005; Satyanarayana, 2007).

Public Health and Patents

Huge investment, long term research, advance clinical trials, and regularity procedures has made health research activities much complex and expensive. Intellectual Property Rights (IPR), the exclusive legal rights granted for an *invention,* has therefore become one of the major incentives for the researchers as well as investors in health sector.

The patent system is designed to promote innovation and, at the same time, offer a mechanism ensuring that the fruits of that innovation are accessible to society. In the contexts of public health, the challenge for policy makers is to find an optimal balance between the rights of patent owners, who provide technological innovations to improve health conditions, and the needs of the general public.

Clearing issues, such as ownership and licensing policies for innovation derived from public research, would contribute to the promotion of a more effective deployment of public funds and public R&D programmes. At the same time, the patent system also contributes to society by making available patent information, which is freely available to other researchers to further improve existing technologies. With a view to facilitating commercialisation and ensuring access to patented technologies, the patent system is primarily based on conferring an exclusive right, in conjunction with a voluntary licensing mechanism.

On the other hand, some consider that the current patent system does not adequately address public health crises. It is argued that the commercial incentives provided by the patent system are not sufficient to ensure the development of new products in certain areas, for example, in respect of neglected diseases, and those patent rights, which are enforced on the basis of commercial and market-based considerations, prevent access to, or increase prices of essential medicines. Some criticise that the safeguard mechanisms built in the patent system, such as compulsory licenses or research exceptions, are not sufficiently broad to cover existing needs. Because of technology disparity between technology exporting and importing countries, a system that works for the developed countries could not do the same in developing countries. Hence socio-economic circumstances of a country must be considered before framing IPR policies.

What an inventor does, if he thinks, he may have made an innovation? There is no answer for this question in the context of our country. Innovations could be a novel treatment, a new diagnosis, a device, drug, new uses of drugs, data and information, software, training materials, treatment protocols, new management system and so on. Publication is one of the reliable methods of dissemination; however, it does not always protect the innovation of a researcher. Publication, presentation in workshop, seminars, and any kinds of disclosure in public space may lose validity for IPR claims in future.

Challenges to be Met

In the contexts of public health, the challenge for policy makers is to find an optimal balance between the rights of patent owners, who provide technological innovations to improve health conditions, and the needs of the general public. There is a need to undertake mapping of R&D gaps in the Type I, II and III diseases giving emphasis to instances where IPRs have failed to provide incentive for investment into research and development of appropriate health care products. Also it must be ensured that if drugs for Type I diseases are available in a developed country; they should be available in developing countries at reasonable prices. The accessibility and affordability of these drugs in developing countries should be studied and lacunae identified.

Steps by national governments as well as the international community to reduce the cost of innovation is necessary. Companies should adopt transparent and consisting pricing policies, and should work towards reducing prices on a more consistent basis for developing countries. National Pricing Policy Framework (economic benefit of new drugs) should be developed to ensure affordability. For instance, a country may chose to negotiate the price of drugs, while granting marketing approval for such drugs.

Thus government needs to prioritise health care and, given the leverage to determine prices that patents confer, should adopt measures to promote competition and ensure that pricing of medicines is consistent with their public health policies. Access to drugs cannot depend on the decisions of private companies but also is a government responsibility (WHO, 2006).

Encourage the use of traditional medicine with lesser emphasis on protection and a greater focus on benefit to the community that generated the knowledge. A regional data base (of patents granted and patent applications filed) should be generated which could be used by patent examiners to ensure that no frivolous patents are granted. This database could also be used by researchers and policy makers. There is a need to ensure greater transparency in granting of patents. This would facilitate pre- and post-grant opposition and prevent 'frivolous patents'.

Public-Private Partnerships are a central feature of global health landscape. With increasing urbanisation, as collaboration between researchers, both local and international continues to increase, the rights of less influential researchers, may it be local or international to be protected through IPR needs to be looked into seriously. Little is known about the effectiveness of partnerships, lack of transparency in how they operate and what they achieve. Benefits achieved through these collaborations whether effectively shared with the society are ambiguous to predict. Whether the rights and privileges of the local researchers are protected or exploited through IPR is not known. Hence a proper system of institutional governance is required. IPR management is a key but complex issue involving several interrelated activities. The procedure of marketing patented ideas, negotiating contracts and agreements on confidentiality, secrecy and licensing also seeking financial support to secure IPR protection needs to be taken care. Even though there are number of local/private organisations dealing with IPR, their active role in capacity building is negligible. Lawyers and law firms are most useful in assisting various IPR management, protection and infringement of patents in India and abroad, but how many of them are well versed to meet the challenges of new IP regime specific in areas of drug discovery, genomics, health research, nanotechnology etc. need to be addressed.

Another contentious issue in the India–European Union (EU) negotiations is regulation of data protection (RDP). It provides an important complementary IP right to patents, which are already accepted in India. Patents are not always available to protect new medicines where much has been invested to generate regulatory data necessary for authorisation and marketing. RPD is essential to protect this investment for a limited period only regardless of patentability (Shahani, 2011). Absence of RDP is most glaring gap in India's R&D environment.

Overcoming Challenges

Introduction of RDP will end unfairness of a situation where investment in knowledge of the originator can be appropriated by another company without protection or compensation. Its implementation will attract foreign direct investment (FDI) in pharma sector; RDP is especially significant when strong patent protection for specific product is not available and where the patent enforcement systems are inadequate.

It must be understood, that real barrier to access to new medicines is not unaffordable cost but, lack of proper health care financing policy, hence concrete steps need to taken in letter and spirit.

A national IPR guideline need to be framed. It should be developed with the objective of reinforcing the innovation capacity of the country. A properly developed IPR guideline provides entrepreneurship friendly environment for commercial application and participate in the development of products and processes useful to national health programmes.

While India has entered the global patent regime, awareness and expertise on the subject of IPR in India is still inadequate. Present skills do not extend towards protecting indigenous inventions or understanding the implications of patents granted to competitors. Further, the ability to read or write patents is grossly lacking when viewed in the context of global practices. India's knowledge-based industries will be looking at filing international patents and their skills in filing, reading and exploring patents will be very crucial in the years to come. Thus national IP institutes should be set up which will be dedicated to carry on a thorough IP research, setting a national innovative culture and capacity building.

India is well poised to make the transition from generics pharma power house to an innovation giant. But to transform this dream into reality, it needs to put in place proper patent protection policies that enforce IPR laws in the country.

References

Flood, P., M. Heffernan, J. Farrell, S. McCurtain, T. O'Hara, P. Regan, and C. Carroll. 2002. *Managing Knowledge-based Organisations: Top Management Teams and Innovation in the Indigenous Software Industry*. Black Hall Publishing, Dublin.

Harrison, S. and P.H. Sullivan. 2000. Profiting from Intellectual Capital: Learning from Leading Companies. *Journal of Intellectual Capital,* 1 (1): 33–46.

Prahalad, C.K. and G. Hamel. 1990. The Core Competence of the Corporation. *Harvard Business Review,* 68 (3): 79–88.

Richard, G. and H. Matthew. 2007. *OECD International Futures Project on the Bio-economy to 2030: Designing a Policy Agenda*. Report: OECD International Futures Programme.

Saha, R. 2005. *Management of Intellectual Property Rights in India*. <http://www.pfc.org.in/workshop/workshop.pdf>. 14 February 2011.

Satyanarayana, K. 2007. 'Current IP Management Issues for Health and Agriculture in India', in A. Krattiger, R.T. Mahoney, L. Nelson, J.A. Thomson, A.B. Bennett, K. Satyanarayana, G.D. Graft, C.

Fernandez, and S.P. Kovalsky (eds), *Intellectual Property Management in Health and Agricultural Innovation: A Handbook of Best Practices*. MIHR and Davis, PIPRA, Oxford, pp. 1605–20.

Shahani, R. 2011. Its Right Medicine: Recognizing Regulatory Data Protection Will Benefit India's Pharma Industry. *The Times of India,* 6 April 2011.

Straus, J. 2004. 'Intellectual Property and Science: A Complex Partnership', in *ALLEA Biennial Yearbook,* Critical Topics in Science and Scholarship. ALLEA, Amsterdam, pp. 19–28.

World Health Organization. 2006. *Public Health: Innovation and Intellectual Property Rights.* Report of the Commission on Intellectual Property Rights, Innovation and Public Health, World Health Organization, Geneva.

World Intellectual Property Organization. 2004. The Impact of Electronic Commerce on Intellectual Property. Primer on Intellectual Property Issues Related to Electronic Commerce. <http://ecommerce.wipo.int/primer/section3.html>. 14th February 2011.

CHAPTER 3

Mental Health

An Overview

SHYAMAL KUMAR NANDY, SUPURNA DAS AND AMITAVA MUKHERJI

Mental Health

Mental health is a condition to enjoy life in a positive capacity in terms of emotional as well as spiritual well-being. Major emphasis has been given on the importance of socio-cultural phenomena operating within a community because of the fact that the socio-cultural processes act upon the mind of the individual to a great extent. Health has been defined by the World Health Organization (WHO) with a broad canvas covering physical, mental and social well-being wherein mental health is as important as the physical and social health to conceptualise health as a whole.

Mental Illness

Mental illness, on the other hand, is conceptuaiised as the alteration in the thinking process and deviations from the normative behaviour which is a preconditioned state of mind, build up through socio-cultural processes of a community. It is also associated with stress, strain, distress, mood swing as well as impaired functioning of mind. Besides, its symptoms vary according to the types of illnesses within a given socio-cultural environment.

The Continuum Concept

There is a continuum between the state of mental health and the state of mental illness but the point of demarcation is not very clear in between. The clinical psychologists, psychiatrists and social-cultural anthropologists may play their respective roles together to cure the mal-adaptive behaviour of the individuals. The treatment is synthesised mainly in two ways – biologically as well as culturally, but we do not have any specific answer regarding how far only the biological way of treating the mental patients are effective or vice versa. There are some antidepressant, antipsychotic medicines which are effectively used by the psychiatrists to reduce the nature of mal-adaptive behaviour and these work at the individual level. But questions arise whether only the cognitive therapy can cure the mental patients without using the medicines. Besides, how far the social-cultural approach can be effective to reduce the mal-adaptive behaviour is also an important question. "The boundaries between health and disease are far from clear, partly because of the roles played by psychological, social, and cultural factors as well as biological ones. Given the multiple factors that affect people, an extreme organic perspective is likely to be oversimplified. More likely to stand the test of time, is a model that views mal-adaptive behaviour as a product of these interacting factors. Although it does not provide a final answer, the biological perspective has enhanced our understanding of one of these sets of factors" (Sarason and Sarason, 2002). Mental health problems and mental illnesses are not the same thing but prolonged mental health problems lead to the mental illnesses.

Review of Literature

Reviews on some of the earlier studies may shed some light regarding the nature of the mental problems and its manifestations in the form of diseased conditions and illnesses. An important study was conducted by Elwin (1950) among the Maria tribal community, dealing with their problems of suicide. He also reviewed many works on suicide like Fenton (1941), Beech (1915), East (1913), Rose (1922), Steinmetz (1894), etc. Some of the authors have dealt with the suicide cases of the primitive people. He mentioned that the study of the suicide cases in the primitive cultures has been neglected in Indian situation. Although there are some rare cases of suicides among the tribals in general but it is common among the Lhota Naga, but it is rare among other Naga tribes.

In 1936, a committee was formed in New York for ethnological studies of the suicides among the primitive people where it occurred frequently, and had thrown some light on suicide as a psycho-biological phenomena as cited by Elwin (1950) from Medical Review of Reviews, New York. Such kind of studies gained importance and urged by many authors like Laubscher (2003) in South Africa who stated that 'It is generally believed that the rate of suicide increases with civilisation. For this reason, I consider that whatever evidence can be produced about suicide in a primitive culture is of great importance to psychiatry.'

Elwin (1950) contributed in the field of social anthropology based on the studies of crime and suicide of the Maria tribe. In the preface of the book *Maria Murder and Suicide* he has explained the social anthropological viewpoint and provided an example of murder of Tati Hirme by her deceased husband's younger brother, Doga. He explained this apparent meaningless crime with the help of the knowledge of a local custom. He stated:

> According to tribal practice a younger brother has a right over his elder brother's widow, a right which extends not only to her person, but to her property. This right Tati Hirme refused to Doga, and there is evidence that for a long time the youth bitterly resented her behaviour. On the day of the tragedy he went to her house and asked her for some tobacco. She

> refused, and he murdered her. At first sight here is precisely one of those motiveless crimes which have so often puzzled outside observers. It is true that there was hostility between the parties, but the refusal of a small gift of tobacco was hardly sufficient for so disastrous a result. But in Maria practice to ask a woman for tobacco is a symbolic way of inviting her to sexual intercourse, and the boy asked his elder brother's widow to have congress with him, he was only demanding his right and when she refused it, he found the provocation, both to his pride and his desire, so great that he killed her. (Elwin, 1950)

He summarised by saying that 'Research, both by medical sciences and by anthropology, may in time reveal how far the apparently motiveless homicides of aboriginals can be explained as crimes of exhaustion and fatigue'.

Durkheim (1951) observed high rate of suicide caused due to industrialisation and social disorganisation. He used the quantitative method and found different suicide rates among Protestants and Catholics. He was of the opinion that rigid social control among the Catholics was the causative factor for their lower suicide rates.

Elwin (1950) has also touched upon the aspects of the fear of persecution, the blood-feud, disputes about property, crime and alcohol, the attitude of the criminal and the attitude to the criminal of the Bondo tribe, in the chapter on the problem of mal-adjustment, of the book entitled as *Bondo Highlander*. Moreover, there are many more studies in the fields of murder as crime and related punishments therein, along with the causes of crimes and suicides; many of which have dealt with the tribal societies. Notable contribution was made by Malinowski (1926) in his famous book entitled as *Crime and Custom in Savage Society* regarding suicide among the Trobriand Islanders. Malinowski opined,

> It looms large in the psychology of the natives, is a permanent damper on any violence of language or behavior, on any deviation from custom to tradition, which might hurt or offend

another. Thus suicide, like sorcery, is a means of keeping the native to the strict observance of a law, a means of preventing people from extreme and unusual types of behavior. (Cited by Elwin, 1950)

In Indian context, Sachidananda (1957), Gupta (1960), Saran (1974), Rao (1975), Nayak (1989), and many others have contributed significantly in this interesting field of research.

There are many contrasting views regarding the prevalence of mental problems in terms of the rural as well as urban situations. Among them, Wig (1981) advocated the prevalence of severe mental illnesses in Indian situation in comparison to the West. Again, he has viewed the higher incidence in rural situation. Other studies by Larsy (1977), Mahanta (1979) and Ahmad (1999) highlighted the same views and stated that the mental health problems were greater among the people living in remote non-industrial rural areas than the people living close to urban/industrial situation or within it.

Prabhu (1980) not found much variation in the prevalence rates of mental illnesses in rural and urban areas specially in the semi-rural, industrial and non-industrial urban population but also reported that the lower prevalence in the rural areas than in any other areas.

Another study by Ahmad (1999) examined the effect of industrialisation, age as well as religion on the mental health of the Oraon tribal population through some important psychological tests with the help of socio-economic status scale, mental health scale and security-insecurity test. He collected data from the Oraon employees of the Heavy Engineering Corporation of Ranchi and also from the Oraon cultivators of the adjacent villages, to which Oraon employees originally belonged. He concluded from this study that the impact of industrialisation had not caused any significant effect on the mental health of the studied Oraon tribal community in general. Religion was found as the main causative factor for the mental health problems rather than other factors like industrialisation and age. This study also revealed that 'the Christians of the industrial area found to be more secure as compared to the Christian of non-industrial area. Age has also been found producing its effect with religion and industrialisation. Young non-Christians from industrial areas and young Christians from non-industrial areas tend to show higher degree of insecurity than their counter parts belonging to the old age-group' (Ahmad, 2010).

On the other hand, Mclean and Taylor (1958) estimated severe mental health problems within industrial workers which varied nearly 15 to 85 per cent. Bhaskaran et al. (1970) also found the same type of scenario among the population living in the industrial situation in comparison to the non-industrial situation. It was also noticed that the people living in the area of culture contact have more anxiety and frustration (Gulati, 1982).

To find out the right scenario of the mental health problems in rural and urban situations, the methodological orientations may differ because of the fact that 'the rural and urban constitute two largely independent subsystems which require separate tools for data collection, and separate parameters for analysis and understanding in their own right. Data and models of this urban discipline provide inadequate basis for understanding rural culture and behaviour. The core characteristics of rural environment make it qualitatively distinct from the urban and any analysis of rural life has to be done against its own backdrop' (Sinha, 1985).

There are some community-based studies conducted in rural areas. Nandi et al. (1975, 1976) studied 1060 individuals from an extremely backward village of West Bengal mainly inhabited by the poor Muslim agriculturalists. Interestingly, they found that in 77 families, out of 177 families studied, at least one person was mentally ill. They also reported that the affected members were from big families and very common symptoms were anxiety, epilepsy, depression, and hysteria. Later they studied the same village population and calculated rates of various types of mental illnesses. The rate of depression in that population was 4.63/1000 and the rate of schizophrenia was

0.93/1000. This study was unique for its approach in the population of a rural area. Surya et al. (1964) did not find even a single case of depression in their survey conducted in Pondicherry. Carstairs (1958) reported only one case of depression in a Rajasthan village. These findings are too old to understand the mental health situation at present in terms of the incidence rate. Varma (1973) mentioned the increase of mental illness since 1959 on the basis of hospital data among the tribals. His study mentioned that schizophrenia was common among the tribals as among the non-tribal population in that area. He also stated that there were significantly high rate of alcoholic psychoses, epilepsy, toxic psychoses, mental sub-normality and cerebral arteriosclerosis among the tribals.

The importance of the rural community based studies focusing on the roles and relations of the community members and the family as well in terms of the mental health problems and its causes and consequences are gaining momentum both in India and abroad (Sinha, 1988). The culture specific study has also been made through rituals (Chakraborty and Banerji, 1975) to ascertain neurosis and obsessional state in Bengali culture.

Many interesting aspects have come up from the foregoing reviews. The socio-economic and socio-cultural factors are also contributing to the prevalence of mental illnesses such as economic stress, problems within the family, forced marriages, cultural values in terms of any kind of restrictions and many other factors with the society. Such aspects have been touched upon by many researchers to find out the genesis of the problem of mental illness at present and earlier also. The emphasis is directed towards the lifestyle oriented activities at the individual level as well as in the structural family therapy (Nandy, 2011) to ameliorate the prevalence of mental illnesses.

The Role of Social Support

Some researchers have worked extensively on the role of social support as an indicator for the reduction of stress and promoter of mental health. The social support system at the family as well as community level is decreasing day-by-day, due to the fragmentation of the traditional joint family system. The increasing number of nuclear families are unable to give proper social support in the sense that the nuclear family members are very busy in their other sphere of activities rather than be attentive to their family members and their day-to-day problems. This situation prevails at present in many families mainly residing in urban areas.

The nature of role and relation have changed to a great extent at the family as well as community level. The nuclear family members at present are found to depend on the friendship for social support to cope with the situation, but that kind of dependence is not in a position to socially support them fully as they used to get from earlier joint family and community set up. Questions on how can we get social support in case of any stressful situation are arising in front of us. 'Even vulnerable people who feel that they are accepted and valued by others are more likely to cope well with stress and are less likely to develop maladaptive symptoms. In addition, their work focuses attention on prevention and ways in which communities can become more supportive places to live' (Sarason and Sarason, 2002).

Renowned actor Kabir Bedi's narrative is mentioned here to feel the situation which is no doubt painful but an eye-opener.

> In the case of my son Siddhartha, it was a completely different experience. He was suffering from Schizophrenia, a tragic condition that affects young adults. Medicine can only control and subdue it; there is no concept of a complete cure. He committed suicide because he felt that there is no light at the end of his tunnel of problems. He felt that he would have lived the drugged existence (in medical terms) and be dysfunctional for the rest of his life. Nothing made sense to his mind. Food felt tasteless, colours meant nothing – for him life was all grey. It was a conscious decision. We knew he was contemplating suicide and we talked him out of it. We called

a suicide prevention centre in California. They came and talked to him but he still went ahead and did it. (*The Asian Age*, 28 March 2010)

An Approach to the Study of Mental Health Problems

It is generally observed that the mental patients are coming to a clinic mainly from the urban and semi-urban areas in and around Kolkata and the number of patients are increasing day-by-day. This observation is significant in terms of the idea that urban population is affected more in number by mental disorders than the rural population, due to complex nature of socio-economic situation in the urban areas.

An examination of the mental health status of the people living in rural area in general and mentally-ill in particular may throw some light here to find out the correlation between the demographic and other cultural variables. The cultural attributes of the studied individuals may also be examined in terms of personal as well as collective habits and practices like performance of meditation and prayer (*japa-tapa*), inclination towards any kind of religious beliefs and practices, nature of passing the leisure time within and outside the community set up, collective exchanges and sharing of thoughts and the like.

Some of the cultural attributes are formally practiced within the family and some others are performed within the community – like playing games in the club or in the courtyard of the village school or in the common place where many people are assembled mainly on a holiday. Such cultural activities give a chance to a person to interact with other members of the community and exchange information or friendship-based gossiping which helps to the bonding of two or more minds. As a social animal, human beings cannot stay for a long time without talking.

We can observe human health physically and perceive its nature to some extent but cannot observe human mind. Thinking processes which are manifested through attitude and behaviour of human beings could be governed by the cultural attributes of a particular society. It is also expressed through dialect by which we can perceive human mind to a great extent. Every culture has its own in-built mechanism which helps to maintain the balance of human mind at its optimum level, in terms of adjustment in emotion and behaviour as a whole through collective performance or some performances in the psychological state of human mind. It is generally stated that the human mind has got the inherent power of adjustment. That power, sometimes, is shattered through anger, agitation, sorrow or any kind of displeasure or by any kind of events in the course of life. Some may overcome problems of life but others may not succeed. It is an ongoing process of adjustment within the psyche to feel comfortable and a process of feeling of satisfaction among others. But any kind of deviation from the normative behaviour of any human being are expressed in their attitudinal perspective, and too much deviation for a long period of time may affect the well-being of the mental health and needs psychiatric attention for maintaining bio-chemical imbalances through medication.

It seems that anthropologists may play an effective role to ascertain the mental problems at the family and community level through participatory studies or otherwise in the wider social perspective for the betterment of interactive communication at the informal level through open ended dialogue. In this regard, anthropologists may join hands with the psychologists to study the mental health status and any kind of deviations therein through intensive fieldwork with a view to find out the inherent in-built mechanisms which are operating at the community level, if any, and how these mechanisms are operating to maintain the mental health. It is only a conceptual exposition for further micro-level understanding of the nature of mental health-status through intensive fieldwork.

References

Ahmad, S.I. 1999. *Industrialization and Mental Health: An Ethno-psychological Study*. Anthropological Survey of India, Kolkata.

Beech, Mervyn W.H. 1915. Suicide amongst the A-Kikuyu of East Africa. *Man*, 13 (30): 56–57.

Bhaskaran, K.B., B.C. Seth and S.N. Yadav. 1970. Migration and Mental Illhealth in Industry. *Indian Journal of Psychiatry*, 12: 102–16.

Carstairs, G.M. 1958. Some Problems of Psychiatry in Patients from Alien Cultures. *Lancet*, 1: 1217–19.

Chakraborty, A. and G. Banerji. 1975. Ritual, a Culture Specific Neurosis and Obsessional States in Bengali Culture. *Indian Journal of Psychiatry*, 17: 273–80.

Durkheim, E. 1897 (1951). *Suicide: A Study in Society*. The Free Press, New York.

East, W.N. 1913. On Attempted Suicide, with an Analysis of 1,000 Consecutive Cases. *Journal of the Mental Science*, 59: 428–78.

Elwin, Verrier. (1943) 1950. *Maria Murder and Suicide*. Oxford University Press, London.

Fenton, W.N. 1941. *Iroquois Suicide: A Study in the Stability in a Culture Pattern*. Smithsonian Institution Bureau of American Ethnology, Bulletin no. 128, Anthropological Papers no. 14, US Govt. Printing Office, Washington DC, p: 134.

Gulati, R.K. 1982. Impact of Development of Science and Technology on the Environment of Tribal Life. *Vanyajati*, 30: 3–7.

Gupta, R.K. 1960. Witchcraft Murders in Duars. *Man in India*, 40 (4): 309–19.

Lasry, J.C. 1977. Cross-cultural Perspective on Mental Health and Immigrant Adaptation. *Social Psychiatry*, 12: 49–55.

Laubscher, L.R. 2003. Suicide in a South African Town: A Cultural Psychological Investigations. *South African Journal of Psychology*, 33(3): 133–43.

Mahanta, J. 1979. *Mental Health and Achievement Motivation of Juang Tribe in Changing Socio-cultural Setting*. Unpublished Ph.D. Thesis, Utkal University, Bhubaneswar.

Malinowski, B. 1926. *Crime and Custom in Savage Society*. Routledge and Kegan Paul Ltd, London.

Mclean, A.A. and G.C. Taylor. 1958. *Mental Health in Industry*. McGraw-Hill Book Company, New York.

Nandi, D.N., S. Ajmany, H. Ganguli, G. Banerjee, G.C. Boral, A. Gosh, and S. Sarkar. 1975. Psychiatric Disorders in a Rural Community in West Bengal: An Epidemiological Study. *Indian Journal of Psychiatry*, 17: 87–99.

——. 1976. The Incidence of Mental Disorders in One Year in a Rural Community in West Bengal. *Indian Journal of Psychiatry*, 18: 79–87.

Nandy, S.K. 2011. The Role of Family in Mental Health and Illness: An Anthropological Viewpoint. *Journal of the Anthropological Survey of India*, 60: 102–7.

Nayak, P.K. 1989. *Blood, Women and Territory: An Analysis of Clan Feuds of Dongria Kondhs*. Reliance Publishing House, New Delhi.

Prabhu, G.G. 1980. 'Deviance and Pathology', in Udai Pareek (ed.), *A Survey of Research in Psychology, 1971–1976, Part I*, Popular Prakashan, Bombay.

Rao, A.V. 1975. 'Suicide in India', in N.L. Faberow (ed.), *Suicide in Different Cultures*. University Park Press, Baltimore.

Rose, H.J. 1922. 'Suicide', in James Hastings (ed.), *Encyclopedia of Religion and Ethics, Vol. XII*. Charles Scribner's Sons, New York.

Sachidananda. 1957. Crime and Punishment in a Munda Village. *Man in India*, 37 (2): 124–32.

Saran, A.C. 1974. *Murder and Suicide among the Munda and the Oraon*. National Publishing House, New Delhi.

Sarason, I.G. and B.R. Sarason. 2002. *Abnormal Psychology: The Problem of Maladaptive Behavior* (10th Edition). Pearson Education Asia, New Delhi.

Sinha, D. 1985. 'Psychology in Rural Areas: The Case of a Developing Country', in R. Diaz-Guerrero (ed.), *Cross-Cultural and National Studies in Social Psychology*. Elsevier Science Publishers, Amsterdam.

Sinha, D. 1988. 'The Family Scenario of a Developing Country and Its Implications for Mental Health: The Case of India', in P.R. Dasan, J.W. Berry and N. Sartorius (eds), *Health and Cross-Cultural Psychology: Towards Applications*. Sage, Newbury Park, California.

Steinmetz, S.R. 1894. Suicide among Primitive Peoples. *American Anthropologist*, 7 (1): 53–60.

Surya, N.C., S.P. Datta, R. Gopalakrishna, D. Sundaram, and J. Kutty. 1964. Mental Morbidity in Pondicherry (1962–1963). *Transactions of All India Institute of Mental Health*, 4: 50–56.

The Asian Age. 2010. The Age on Sunday-Hertitude. *The Asian Age*, 28 March 2010, p. 19.

Varma, L.P. 1973. Mental Disorders among the Adivasis. *Journal of Clinical Psychiatry*, 1: 21–29.

Wig, N.N. 1981. Incidence of Severe Mental Illness in India: No Less Than West. *Medical Times*, 1: 1.

CHAPTER 4

Mega Urbanisation and Plant Genetic Erosion

BINI TOMS

Introduction

Today, human activities and race for industrialisation, modernisation and scientific developments have lead to erosion of plant genetic resources. If we look back, history offers countless examples of the dependence of human beings on plants for survival. We are aware of instances of the development of treatments and vaccines from plant sources when diseases and pandemics have struck the human race unaware. Moreover, loss of biodiversity is one of the seven indicators of unacceptable environmental changes and therefore, to ensure human health and survival, conservation of plant genetic resources and maintaining the plant gene pool is vital. In this chapter, I will explain how plant genetic erosion affects human health; explore reasons for the increasing erosion and ways to address the issue.

Scope

The issue of increasing plant genetic erosion due to mega urbanisation, its impact on human health and ways to address the issue are discussed under the following heads:

- Definition of Plant Genetic Erosion and Extent
- Definition of Human Health
- The Connection between Plant Genetic Erosion and Human Health
- Plant Genetic Erosion: Reasons and Concerns
- Addressing the Concerns

Definition of Plant Genetic Erosion and Extent

Let me begin by defining and explaining the term plant genetic erosion. In general terms 'biodiversity' means 'variety of life'. For biologists, 'biodiversity' refers to the quantity of species and the variety of environments in which species or genes are present. 'Genetic erosion' is defined as the loss of genetic diversity and commonly refers to the reduction in the quantities of specimens of a species (Solbrig, 1991).

For agricultural crops, however, genetic erosion occurs not just by the reduction in the number of plants of a species or in the geographic range of a species, but, more importantly, the loss of genetic variation among the plants, or more precisely, the loss of some of the diverse forms of genes (i.e., alleles) that are the primary source of the variation in appearance and in the life cycles of plants.

According to Michael (1998), it also means the loss of genetic information that occurs when highly adaptable cultivars are developed and threaten the survival of their more locally adapted ancestors, which form the genetic base of the crop. For example, a new hybrid strain of maize (*Zea mays*), developed largely by Donald F. Jones from a variety discovered in 1917, had yields 25 per cent greater than standard maize. By the 1960s it was economically very favourable to use this single hybrid type, and more traditional varieties rapidly receded in distribution. The widespread adoption of this hybrid led to the narrowing of the genetic base (i.e., genetic erosion). In 1962 workers in the Philippines noticed that the fungus *Helminthosporium maydis* (southern corn leaf blight) was highly virulent on this hybrid. By 1970, 80 per cent of the US crop was vulnerable to *Helminthosporium maydis ions*, because of the heavy dependence on the one hybrid, and during the wet summer of 1970 around 20 per cent of the US crop was lost to the blight. Fortunately, in this case the genetic resources needed to produce a resistant strain had not become completely obsolete and so a recovery could be made.

Having defined the term it is important to discuss whether plant genetic erosion is really taking place. If yes, at what rate? Let us look at just a few examples of plant genetic erosion which would give us an idea of the extent of erosion.

Examples of Genetic Erosion

- A survey of far household in the Republic of Korea showed that of 14 crops cultivated in home gardens, an average of only 26 per cent of the land cultivated there in 1985, were still present in 1993.
- In China, in 1949, nearly 10,000 wheat varieties were used in production. By the 1970s, only about 1,000 varieties remained in use.
- In Malaysia, the Philippines and Thailand it is reported that local fruit varieties are gradually being replaced with modern varieties.
- In Ethiopia, traditional barley and durum wheat varieties are suffering serious genetic erosion due to displacement by introduced varieties.
- Large-scale genetic erosion of local varieties of native Andean crops is reported in Equador and Argentina.
- Chile reports genetic erosion of local potato varieties as well as other crops such as oats, barley, lentils, watermelon, tomato, and wheat.
- Only 20 per cent of the local maize varieties cultivated in 1930 are now known in Mexico.

Source: (Friss-Hansen, 1999)

These are just few examples. The problem has affected the whole world. In 2005, Conservation International has identified

34 hotspots which cover 2.3 per cent of the earth's land surface, yet more than 50 per cent of the world's plant species and 42 per cent of all terrestrial vertebrate species are endemic to these areas. All are threatened by human activities. 'With limited funding and an inadequate number of scientists, governments in countries containing hotspots of threatened biodiversity are wrestling with how to protect plants and animals in disappearing habitats' (Sanders, 2009).

Definition of Human Health

Would the present rate of plant genetic erosion have impact on human kind? In other words, is it a relevant issue for discussion in human health research context? To answer the question we need to look at the definition of human health.

The term health has a range of meanings and associated methods of measurement. Perhaps the most familiar of these is the medical and health care view of health as the absence of disease. Medical indicators thus measure health through factors such as infant mortality, life expectancy and the incidence of diseases such as coronary heart disease and cancer. Defining health in this way has commonly been referred to as a negative definition. However, over the past decade or so there has been a shift in the meaning of the term 'health'. The trend is towards broadening the definition and taking a more holistic definition. The WHO defines health as 'a state of complete physical, mental and social well-being and not merely the absence of disease...' WHO's Ottawa charter defines it as 'a concept for everyday life, emphasising social – peace, shelter, education, food, income, a stable ecosystem, sustainable resources, social justice, equity, and personal physiologic resources.

The Connection between Plant Genetic Erosion and Human Health

In the late 1990s a model of health determinants came up which was advanced with further research into details of the social factors (Barton et al., 2003). This ecosystem model of a neighbourhood indicates the interrelationship between people's health and their neighbourhood. It shows that community and healthy activities can be supported or frustrated by the form of the built environment, as can the relationships between people and natural resources. It suggests that health is not only the concern of the health sector. According to Stott, 80 per cent of our health is determined by policies and activities outside the health sector (Brown and Grant, 2005).

Our discussion leads us to the thought that there is a need for biodiversity conservation. This model emphasises the connection between biodiversity conservation and human health status which further strengthens our point about the need of conservation. In fact, there is more than one argument in favour of preserving biodiversity and maintaining healthy ecosystems. According to the national geographic expeditions, 2008 the five major categories of these arguments are as follows:

- *Economic:* 'Biodiversity can help people make money or keep people from losing money.'
- *Recreational:* 'People love outdoor activities like fishing and backpacking, which would not be possible if ecosystems were destroyed.'
- *Cure:* 'Biodiversity can help people find better cures for illnesses.'
- *Human rights:* 'If biodiversity is protected, indigenous people can continue to live in their native lands.'
- *Spiritual:* 'Biodiversity should be preserved for its own sake;' 'Animals and plants have a right to live;' and 'People rely on wild places and creatures for spiritual fulfillment.'

Plant Genetic Erosion: Reasons and Concerns

Loss of biodiversity has also been recognised as one of the seven indicators of unacceptable environmental changes (Rockström et al., 2009) and therefore, conservation of plant genetic diversity is extremely important. The new Copenhagen accord also recognises that climate change is one of the greatest challenges of the present and that actions should be taken to keep any temperature rises to below 2°C (BBC News, 2009). However, steps for plant genetic biodiversity conservation were neither addressed at this international conference nor are it sufficiently discussed in scientific circles. The conference discussed just one issue related to plant biodiversity conservation and that is, the reduction of deforestation in return for cash from developed countries (John et al., 2009).

Besides the role of plants in maintaining ecological balance, history offers countless examples of the dependence of human beings on plants for survival. We are aware of instances of the development of treatments and vaccines from plant sources when diseases and pandemics have struck the human race unaware. According to the World Health Organization, plant medicines, today, account for over $60 billion in sales worldwide. In the United States, the sources of 40 per cent of medicines are plants and 80 per cent of the world's population uses herbs as their primary medicines (Kilham, 2009). The list of plant-derived vaccinogens continues to grow (Walmsley and Arntzen, 2000). Therefore, to ensure human health and survival, conservation of plant genetic resources and maintaining the plant gene pool is vital.

Moreover, improved agricultural practices and industrialisation are resulting in growing genetic erosion of plant resources as discussed in the next section. For example, there are just 150 crops which feed the people on this planet today as compared to 10,000 plant species at the dawn of agriculture (FAO, 2004). Thus, plant diversity conservation is a necessity today. In addition, plant diseases and abiotic stresses due to climatic changes also threaten us of plant genetic erosion. This threat requires us to work for the production of new types of plant for which the presence of conserved plant genetic diversity and variability is a prerequisite. To put it in another way, good plant gene banks (sources of diverse conserved types of plant) are the only sources for gene hunters working for improvement of agriculture and health care. With global warming and climatic changes threatening that a different ecosystem may arise in a

4°C world (Barnett, 2009; Heffernan, 2009), conservation of each type of plant is even more important as these may be sources of valuable genes. Unfortunately, this important issue has been ignored for a while now.

To stress the importance of plant biodiversity conservation attention towards recent studies with respect to the diversity of human population is drawn. Studies indicate the existence of human phenotypic diversity even within isogenic population of human cells and the scientific opportunities of this field of the study of diversity termed as 'the biology of noise' (Lahn and Ebenstein, 2009; McCullagh et al., 2009). A similar diversity may be expected in plants too, reinforcing the fact that each plant type may be valuable and needs to be conserved. Probably, we need to give importance to a new field, 'bioethics and plant noise conservation' (where noise means genetic diversity) for the good of medical and agricultural research, global health, individuals, the environment and society.

Surprisingly, there are limited guidelines in the world for plant diversity conservation. Moreover, the existing ones are not strictly adhered to. A global document on plant diversity conservation is 'The International Treaty on Plant Genetic Resources for Food and Agriculture', which came into effect on 29 June 2004. The salient points of this treaty include recognising the contribution of farmers to the diversity of crops that feed the world; establishing a global system to provide farmers, plant breeders and scientists with access to plant genetic materials and ensuring benefit sharing (FAO, 2004). In addition, the importance of international cooperation and open exchange of genetic resources for food security is stressed in the treaty. However, the treaty does not talk about the conservation of plant genetic diversity. Another international document on diversity conservation is the Convention on Biological Diversity (CBD) which is discussed later.

So far genetic erosion and its extent, the broad definition of human health and the impact of genetic erosion on human health suggesting the need for plant biodiversity conservation is discussed. Figure 1 below summarises the impact of plant genetic erosion on human health and highlights various human activities which contributes to it.

Figure 1

Impact of Plant Genetic Erosion on Human Health

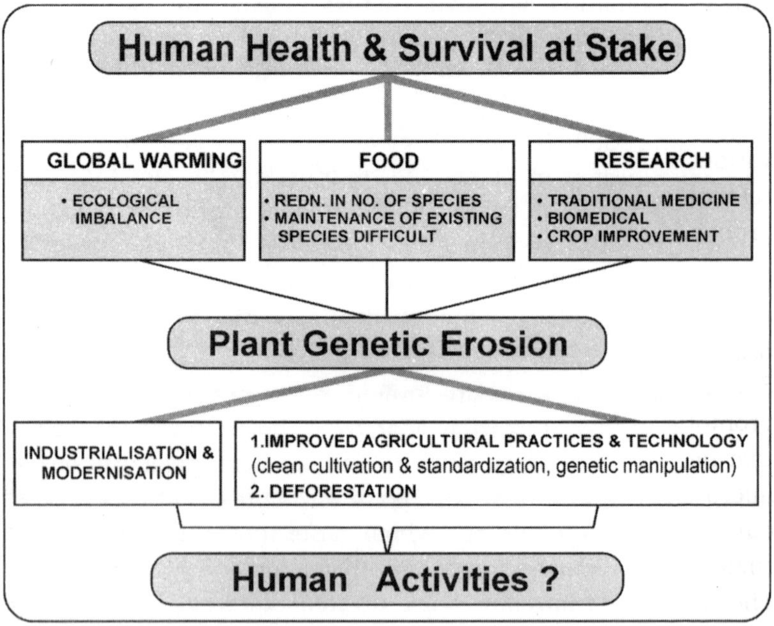

The above figure of human activities have led to a scenario – the glimpse of which is as follows:

- The average temperature of the last 15 years has been the highest ever;
- The icecap is 40 per cent thinner than 40 years ago;
- Over 50 per cent of grain traded all over the world is treated as bio fuels;
- 40 per cent of arable land has suffered long term damage;
- 13 million hectares of forests have disappeared;
- The world spends 12 times more on military expenditures than on helping the poor and downtrodden; and

- One billion people have no access to safe drinking water.

The situation indeed is of grave concern and needs immediate attention. An effort for plant genetic conservation is the need of the hour.

Addressing the Concerns

Initiatives have been taken by different countries (Bertrand, 2009). The movie entitled *Home,* directed by Bertrand, beautifully demonstrates what we are now doing to combat and reverse the damage done: including renewable energy, the creation of more and more national parks, international co-operation between various nations on environmental issues and the education and reforms being initiated across the globe in response to the current problems facing the earth.

As mentioned, an international initiative for biodiversity conservation is the Convention on Biological Diversity (CBD). Signed by 150 government leaders at the 1992 Rio Earth Summit, the Convention on Biological Diversity is dedicated to promoting sustainable development. The Convention recognises that biological diversity is about more than plants, animals and micro organisms and their ecosystems – it is about people and our need for food security, medicines, fresh air and water, shelter, and a clean and healthy environment in which to live. The United Nations proclaimed 22 May of every year as the International Day for Biological Diversity (IDB) to increase understanding and awareness of biodiversity issues. Another international body, the Food and Agriculture Organisation (FAO), works closely with the Convention secretariat on many issues, including joint management of a programme on agricultural biodiversity that draws upon the full range of FAO technical expertise.

In summary, the steps that need to be taken immediately to address the concerns are enlisted below.

- Conservation of all plant types

- Protection of natural habitats
- Avoiding deforestation
- Advocating reforestation and afforestation
- Allocation of funds for conservation
- Wise use of technologies-slow down
- Management of industrialisation
- Public awareness
- Formation and implementation of policies/guidelines

With these doable options available, hope is to check the adverse effects of mega urbanisation, control plant genetic erosion, maintain ecological balance, save earth's vanishing medicine cabinet, ensure continuing health research, and maintain human health on this planet which is home to all.

Conclusion

Indeed, the issue of plant genetic diversity conservation has been ignored for a while. As we contemplate on the major challenges due to mega urbanisation, we need to give a thought to the issue of plant genetic diversity conservation because diversity loss is one of the most important factors contributing to unacceptable climatic changes and global warming (Rockström et al., 2009). The combined efforts of plant scientists, governments and the general public as a whole in this direction is the need of the hour before we are caught in the grip of irreversible loss of plant genetic biodiversity. As Chief Seattle, 1854 has rightly said, 'Man did not weave the web of life; he is merely a strand in it. Whatever he does to the web, he does to himself.'

Acknowledgements: I would like to express my sincere thanks to Dr Nandini K. Kumar and Dr Jerome Singh for their advice and valuable inputs for this write up. I am grateful to Dr Dena Taylor and Jennifer Wilson for their suggestions. I acknowledge NIH for the Fogarty fellowship and the Joint Centre for Bioethics, U of T for its constant support during the course of compilation of this material.

References

Barnett, Anna. 2009. No Easy Way Out (News feature), Nature Reports *Climate Change*, 3 (November): 128–29.

Barton, H., M. Grant and R. Guise. 2003. *Shaping Neighbourhoods*, Spon, London.

BBC News. 2009. *Copenhagen Deal: Key Points.* <http://news.bbc.co.uk/1/hi/sci/tech/8422307.stm> (accessed on 20 December 2009).

Bertrand, Yann Arthus. 2009. *Home*, movie released on 5 June 2009. Produced by Denis Carot and Luc Besson and distributed by Europa Corp., with sponsorship from PPR.

Brown, Caroline and Grant Marcus. 2005. Biodiversity and Human Health: What Role for Nature in Healthy Urban Planning? *Atypon*, 31 (4): 326–38.

Food and Agriculture Organisation. 2004. *International Treaty on Plant Genetic Resources for Food and Agriculture.* www.fao.org/Legal/TREATIES/033s-e.htm (accessed on 19 December 2009).

Friss-Hansen, Esbern. 1999. Erosion of Plant Genetic Resources: Causes and Effects. *Geografisk Tidsskrift, Danish Journal of Geography*, Special Issue 1: 61–68.

Heffernan, Olive. 2009. A Safe Space (Editorial), Nature Reports *Climate Change*, 3 (October): 109.

John, Vidal, Allegra Stratton and Suzanne Goldenberg. 2009. Low Targets, Goals Dropped: Copenhagen Ends in Failure. *The Guardian*, 19 December.

Kilham, Chris. 2009. Plants: The World's Primary Medicines. *Fox News, Health Blog*, 16 September, 2: 09 PM Eastern.

Lahn, Bruce T. and Ebenstein Lanny. 2009. Let's Celebrate Human Genetic Diversity. Opinion, *Nature*, 461: 726–28.

McCullagh, Emma, Justin Farlow, Christopher Fuller, Juliet Girard, Joanna Lipinski-Kruszka, Dan Lu, Thomas Noriega, Geoffrey Rollins, Russell Spitzer, Michael Todhunter, and Hana El-Samad. 2009. Not All Quiet on the Noise Front. *Nature Chemical Biology*, 5 (10): 699–704.

Michael, Allaby. 1998. Genetic Erosion, in *A Dictionary of Plant Sciences*. <http://www encyclopedia.com> (accessed on 27 January 2010).

Rockström, Johan, Will Steffen, Kevin Noone, Åsa Persson, F. Stuart Chapin, Eric F. Lambin, Timothy M. Lenton, Marten Scheffer, Carl Folke, Hans Joachim Schellnhuber, Björn Nykvist, Cynthia A. de

Wit, Terry Hughes, Sander van der Leeuw, Henning Rodhe, Sverker Sörlin, Peter K. Snyder, Robert Costanza, Uno Svedin, Malin Falkenmark, Louise Karlberg, Robert W. Corell, Victoria J. Fabry, James Hansen, Brian Walker, Diana Liverman, Katherine Richardson, Paul Crutzen, and Jonathan A. Foley. 2009. A Safe Operating Space for Humanity. *Nature,* 461: 472–75.

Sanders, Rober. 2009. Predicting Diversity within Hotspots to Enhance Conservation. Media Relations, UC Berkeley news, News Centre, Press Release, 5 February .

Solbrig, O.T. 1991. Ecosystems and Global Environmental Change, in R.W. Corell and P.A. Anderson (eds), *Global Environmental Change*. Springer-Verlag, Berlin, pp. 97–108.

Walmsley, Amanda, M. and J. Arntzen Charles. 2000. Plants for Delivery of Edible Vaccines. *Current Opinion in Biotechnology,* 11 (2): 126–29.

CHAPTER 5

Health and Educational Rights of the Children in an Urban Slum

A Case Study in Dibrugarh District, Assam

PRANJAL BORUAH

India has the largest child population in the world with more than one third of its population below the age of 18 years. The Constitution of India provided for the well-being of children way back in 1950. The National Policy of Children formulated by the Government of India in 1974 described children as 'Supremely important asset'. The convention on the rights of the child, drafted by the UN Commission on Human Rights and adopted by the General Assembly of the United Nations in 1989, is a set of international standards and measures intended to protect and promote the well-being of children in society which was ratified by our country in 1992.

The right to nutrition receives its fullest expression in the 1989 convention on the rights of the child, under which virtually every government in the world recognises the right of all children to the highest attainable standard of health, including the right to good nutrition and its three vital components: food, health and care (Mishra et al., 2001). Despite these efforts, it has been observed that the status of children in India indicates a huge gap between policies and practice.

Over the past five decades India's urban population has increased manyfolds. The recent rapid urban population growth and relative lack of attention to urban poverty has possibly exacerbated deprivation in urban areas. Due to poverty, population explosion and environmental degradation in India, the children of the families below poverty line are mostly deprived from their health and educational rights.

The National Sample Survey of India showed that the urban population below poverty line increased from 60 million in 1973–74 to 80.8 millions in 2004–05 (Tsujita, 2009). With rapid urbanisation and having one of the highest growth rates in the world, around 20 per cent of urban population is forced to reside in urban slums (Mishra et al., 2001). There is a constant deprivation, particularly of the children among these urban poor.

In the present chapter, therefore, an attempt has been made to bring out the health and educational standard of the children among a migrant Muslim community (*Jolah*) inhabiting slums area in Dibrugarh town, Assam.

The National Sample Survey Organization (NSSO), India defines a slum as a 'compact settlement with a collection of poorly built tenements, mostly of temporary nature, crowded together usually with inadequate sanitary and drinking water facilities in unhygienic conditions' (cited in Chandrasekhar, 2005). There are two kinds of slums: notified and non-notified. Areas notified as slums by the respective municipalities, corporations, local bodies or development authorities are treated as notified slums. A slum is considered as a non-notified slum if at least 20 households lived in that area (ibid.). The present study is a non-notified one as it consists of 20 households. The total population is 108, out of this 62 (57.40%) are male and 46 (42.59%) are female.

Standard anthropological tools were used in the collection of field data. It is based on data collected through semi-structured interviews conducted with heads of the households and women.

Living Condition of the People

The people migrated from Gorakhpur to Dibrugarh town with the hope of better means of livelihood. They are residing on the bank of the river Brahmaputra in Dibrugarh town with poorly built tenements mostly of temporary nature and crowded together. They are living in an unhygienic condition. There is no electricity in their houses and in every small room 4–5 individuals sleep at night. As the hearth is attached with the sleeping room, the smoke coming out from each hearth also affects the people. Besides they have inadequate sanitary and drinking water facilities. As they have only one hand pump for these 20 households, they by and large depend upon the river water. During the rainy season they cannot stay in these houses due to water blocking and they have to stay temporarily on the embankment of the river.

The primary occupation of the males is a quack and the females sell glass bangles visiting door to door in different places. Both husband and wife have to earn for the survival of their family. A few young boys also go for different wage earnings. What they earn is only for their daily consumption. The people wake up early in the morning and get busy with their daily works. All families of each household take rice and a little fried vegetable as morning breakfast and complete their breakfast by 7:30 AM. After that, both the men folk and women folk go separately for their own business. The girls generally stay at home to look after their younger siblings and household chores. The children play outside throughout the day. In the evening all the family members meet together and they complete their dinner by 7.30 PM. Every Friday the males go to the *Mazzid* and all the people keep apart money from their daily earning sources.

Health Status of the Children

Poor health is a chronic problem for slum children. Poor water and sanitary conditions lead to adverse health outcomes in the households living in the slums (Kumar et al., 2003). As the people under study are not getting satisfactory quality of water and adequate sanitary facilities, this lead to sickness, causes diarrhoea and other water borne diseases among their children and adults and also affect the life expectancy.

Due to extreme poverty these slum dwellers are forced to live in the most insanitary and unhygienic conditions. Most of the children are affected by worm infection as they move around bare foot.

Half of all children in India are malnourished, but for slum children the proportion is much higher. The children under study are not only underweight, but their growth is often stunted. Due to poor economic condition they are not getting any nutrients. Some children are seen to take only plain rice to satisfy their hunger.

The Government of India is striving hard to reduce the infant mortality rate by providing a variety of maternal and child health care services. The child care services are mainly focused on the immunisation of children against the six major killer diseases and also to educate the mothers regarding diarrhoea and pneumonia which are dangerous for children, all targeted at reduction of infant mortality. Proper breast feeding and weaning practices, complete and timely coverage of immunisation of the children are the two prime aspects in child care, as they ensure the health and chance of survival of the child (Babu and Rao, 2006).

Approximately 2.5 million infants die every year in India from diseases, which can simply be prevented by immunisation. Immunisation against preventable disease is the central concept of the primary health and reproductive and child health care (Jain and Sharma, 2006). Vaccination is a preventive therapy against various diseases of children. To save a pregnant woman and the child in her womb from Tetanus disease it is necessary to give her two injections of TT vaccine during her pregnancy period.

Immunisation of children under study are not regular. Due to illiteracy, they do not know that to save their children from malignant diseases (tetanus, tuberculosis, diphtheria, whopping cough, polio, and measles) vaccination is a must. They do not even know about the vaccination schedule for pregnant women and for infants. Most of the children suffer from various diseases such as fever, diarrhoea, cough, measles, jaundice, malaria, typhoid etc. In some cases death episodes are also recorded from these diseases. Though all kinds of necessary vaccination are supplied free by the government but the people of this slum area are deprived from it. Except the Intensive Pulse Polio Immunization (IPPI) programmes for Oral Polio Vaccine they are not getting the other free vaccines. Though the District Civil Hospital and Assam Medical College of Dibrugarh are very near to them, they are still deprived from health education programme.

Table1

Place of Delivery

No. of Women	*Place of Delivery*		*Total (%)*
	Home (%)	*Hospital (%)*	
20	60 (68.18)	28 (31.82)	88 (100.00)

Table 2

Infant Mortality

Mothers (No. of Women)	*Total No. of Conception*	*Abortion*	*Still Birth*	*Live Birth*	*Post Birth Death*
20	94	6	6	69	13

Most of the deliveries are carried out at home. Table 1 shows that out of 88 issues, 60 (68.18%) are carried out at home and 28 (31.82%) are carried out at hospital. Infant mortality rate is high among them. Table 2 shows that the total number of conception of the 20 women is 94. Out of this 69 are live birth, 6 still birth, 6 abortion and 13 post birth death. They do not have the knowledge of family planning. It is seen that most of the families have 6–7 children. They think that it will be helpful to increase their race to support their economic condition.

Socio-cultural and economic factors complicate their access to health services. Various studies show that slum dwellers have poorer access to health facilities and hence suffer from poor health outcomes (Kapadia-Kundu and Kanitkar, 2002; Kumar et al., 2003; Sundar and Sharma, 2002). The relation between migration and health is a complex one and it operates in both positive and negative directions on the migrant himself or herself and other members of the family and community (Babu et al., 2010). Generally it is seen that people of this area used to get modern facilities offered by the government but they are neglected for their dwelling place. In medical department they are given prescriptions to purchase medicine but they cannot purchase the medicine themselves due to their poor economic conditions.

Educational Status of the Children

In India, though there is a provision of free and compulsory education system to children but, most of the children are still illiterate. During the present investigation it has been observed that out of the total population of 108, 89.81 per cent are illiterate and 10.19 per cent are literate (Table 3). The parents themselves being illiterate cannot encourage their children for education. Day-by-day their children are deprived from right to education. Girls are the first to be victimised in such families. They are generally engaged to look after the younger siblings and do the household chores.

Table 3

Distribution of the Population by Age, Sex and Level of Education

S No.	Age group (in years)	Illiterate			Literate			Grand Total (%)
		Male (%)	Female (%)	Total (%)	Male (%)	Female (%)	Total (%)	
1	0–4	7 (6.48)	8 (7.40)	15 (13.88)	—	—	—	15 (13.88)
2	5–9	9 (8.33)	5 (4.62)	14 (12.96)	3 (2.77)	1 (0.92)	4 (3.70)	18 (16.66)
3	10–14	15 (13.88)	10 (9.25)	25 (23.14)	4 (3.70)	—	4 (3.70)	29 (26.85)
4	15–19	2 (1.85)	1 (0.92)	3 (2.77)	2 (1.85)	1 (0.92)	3 (2.77)	6 (5.55)
5	20–24	—	1 (0.92)	1 (0.92)	—	—	—	1 (0.92)
6	25–29	1 (0.92)	3 (2.77)	4 (3.70)	—	—	—	4 (3.70)
7	30–34	2 (1.85)	10 (9.25)	12 (11.11)	—	—	—	12 (11.11)
8	35–39	9 (8.33)	5 (4.62)	14 (12.96)	—	—	—	14 (12.96)
9	40–44	6 (5.55)	1 (0.92)	7 (6.48)	—	—	—	7 (6.48)
10	45–49	2 (1.85)	—	2 (1.85)	—	—	—	2 (1.85)
	Total	53 (49.07)	44 (40.74)	97 (89.81)	9 (8.33)	2 (1.85)	11 (10.18)	108 (100.00)

Both men and women have to go to work to survive their family. In the absence of parents all the children pass their lives by playing outside. A few of them go to Madrasa School to have the basic primary education. But as they have to pay ₹ 50 monthly for each child, due to poor economy, the children finally are deprived from their education. Besides this, submitting birth certificate is a must and if they cannot submit, they are not allowed to continue their education.

Sometimes husband refuses to give money from his earning to look after his wife and children. In such situation the woman one and only is responsible for the survival of her entire family members. Whatever she earns, is only of use for their daily consumption and finally the school-going children have to leave their school. In this regard a case has been taken.

Case Study

Khusbu Begum (32 years) has four children. Both she and her husband have to earn for their survival. But her husband refuses to share his earned money with them. Though her children went to school but they discontinued it owing to the economic crisis. As reported by her she was again pregnant for the fifth issue but due to her husband's behaviour she is to go for induced abortion.

Poverty is the primary cause of the crisis of slum children. Poverty dumps a crowd of problems onto a child. Not only do these problems cause immediate suffering, they also conspire to keep the child poor throughout his or her life. In order to survive, a poor child in India is probably forced to sacrifice education and training; without skills the child will, as an adult, remain at the bottom of the economic heap. The government educational scheme like *Sarva Sikhsa Abhiyan* is not reaching in the slum areas. Day-by-day these children are deprived of their educational rights.

Concluding Remarks

Poor availability and poor access to government health services among migrant population are universal. The health treatment and behaviour of health staff is not favourable toward migrant people. The people under study are also exposed to neglect. The common factor that justifies their vulnerability is perhaps the fact that their origin differs from their present urban residence. The difference is not merely limited to the experience of change of space but extends to other experiences of differences in culture, language and people. The vulnerability of the migrants becomes complicated by the combination of factors in the urban area. The people are considered as an outsider and so they are deprived from the government facilities. And ultimately it leads to deprivation of their children from health and educational rights.

Education is an important media for bringing about change in any society. By educating people, their economic and social development can be promoted and backward sections of the society can be brought close to advanced communities (Bairathi, 1991). Women education and employment are considered to be decisive factors for the improvement of family life and steady reduction in fertility. A woman's educational status controls the size of her family and health of her family members. So the local self government like municipality and panchayat should keep notice on these people.

Rural to urban migration has been a major explanation for the dramatic increase in urban population in India. Most prominent characteristic of the urbanisation is the mushrooming growth of slums and squatters. These slum/squatter dwellers are marginalised due to unstructured urban health care services. Though present study is a micro level one but day-by-day the family size of this particular community is increasing so there is an urgent need to see such socio-economically disadvantaged population as a serious issue.

References

Babu, B.V., K.S. Basanta, S. Mishra, and S.K. Kar. 2010. Primary Healthcare Services among a Migrant Indigenous Population Living in an Eastern India City. *Journal of Immigrant and Minority Health*, 12 (1): 53–59.

Babu, M.S. and P.D. Rao. 2006. Child Care among Racha Koyaks: A Tribal Group from Andhra Pradesh. *Man and Life*, 32 (3–4): 67–74.

Bairathi, S. 1991. *Tribal, Culture, Economy and Health*. Rawat Publications, Jaipur.

Chandrasekhar, S. 2005. *Growth of Slums, Availability of Infrastructure and Demographic Outcomes in Slums: Evidence from India*. Paper presented during the session on Urbanisation in Developing Countries at the Population Association of America. <http://www.iussp.org/Activities/wgc-urb/chandrasekhar.pdf>. 12 February 2011.

Jain, A.K. and A.N. Sharma. 2006. Feeding Practices, Child Immunization and Malnutrition Problems among the Traditional Prostitutes of Beria Caste of Sagar District, Madhya Pradesh. *Man and Life,* 32 (3–4): 61–66.

Kapadia-Kundu, N. and T. Kanitkar. 2002. Primary Health Care in Urban Slums. *Economic and Political Weekly,* 21 December, 5086–89.

Kumar, S., K. Shigeo and H. Harada. 2003. Living Environment and Health of Urban Poor: A Study in Mumbai. *Economic and Political Weekly,* 23 August, 3575–86.

Mishra, R. N., C.P. Mishra, P. Sen and T.B. Singh. 2001. Nutritional Status and Dietary Intake of Pre-School Children in Urban Slums of Varanasi. *Indian Journal of Community Medicine,* 26 (2): 90–93.

Sundar, R. and A. Sharma. 2002. Morbidity and Utilisation of Healthcare Services: A Survey of Urban Poor in Delhi and Chennai. *Economic and Political Weekly,* 23 November , 4729–40.

Tsujita, Y. 2009. *Deprivation of Education in Urban Areas: A Basic Profile of Slums Children in Delhi, India*. IDE Discussion paper no 199. Institute of Developing Economies, Chiba.

SECTION II

Occupation and Health: The Challenges

CHAPTER 6

Occupational Health and Psychosocial Stress of the Workers in Construction Industry

GUDDI TIWARY AND P.K. GANGOPADHYAY

Industry plays an important role in building up of a nation. According to the National Classification of Industry (1987), Construction industry is under code 5. About 340 million (roughly 92%) of the workforce is engaged in unorganised sector of which around half of them are from the construction industry (Das, 2007; NCEUS, 2006; Rajasekhar et al., 2009; Ramesh, 2007). To safeguard the benefits of the workers and their health, the central and state governments in India have enacted various acts and rules respectively (NCEUS, 2006).The Buildings and Other Construction Workers (regulation of employment and conditions of service) Act, 1996 was enacted by parliament in 1996: the Act regulate the employment and condition of service of buildings and other construction workers and to provide for their safety, health and welfare measures and for other matters connected therewith or incidental thereto (Ministry of Labour and

Employment, GOI, 1996). The maximum stipulated hours of work by Factories Act 1948 is eight hours per day (Sarkar, 2008), but the workers are working 10–12 hours (Lakhani, 2004).

Objectives

The study is aimed to know socio-economic status and health problems of the workers. The different social security measures and schemes for the workers are also seen.

- The socio-economic status and psychosocial stresses of the construction workers of unorganized/informal sector is to be known.
- The different health problems faced by the worker are to be observed.
- The different social welfare measures are to be discussed.

Methodology

Various literatures available regarding different aspects of construction workers have been searched through library and internet. The original literatures available for the last 30 years (papers, book, articles etc.) have been consulted. The salient features have been noted in the different aspects.

Literature Review

Socio-economic Status

In India, 22.68 million of work forces are engaged in construction industry, out of this 18.25 million are casual workers (Fernandes and Paul, 2011; NSSO, 2008). As per Census of India (2001), West Bengal alone covers 864,180 construction workers of which 827,910 are males and 36,270 are females.

The workers are poor and belong from a poor economic background. With so much of hardship they cannot fulfil their daily need of food, clothes, education etc. The workers are poorly paid. It is interesting to note that in 2004, construction industry workers were paid ₹ 76.40 (Chakrabarti, 2005). Revised minimal wage of a construction industry unskilled worker in 2009 is ₹ 179 in Kerala followed by Andaman and Nicobar (₹ 167), Delhi (₹ 152), Haryana (₹ 151) and Chandigarh (₹ 148) (Paycheck India, 2009). West Bengal has ₹ 114 for unskilled workers (Paycheck India, 2009). Average women workers at certain point of time are jobless, getting lesser wage than men (Rajawat, 2003; SEWA, 2000).

Psychosocial Stress

It was also suggested that there was stress due to work burden, repetitive work and job uncertainty (Cox et al., 1979; Malenfant et al., 2007). Psychological ill health is also common with high rates of alcohol and drug abuse (Rothan, 1985; Snashall, 2007). The workers misuse their money on alcohol as they do not have any other recreation. Too much intake of alcohol loses their mental state. This results in beating of wife and children and scolding them for not being able to fulfil their basic needs (food, clothes, education etc.). The nature of work leads to fatigue. Monotonous work, work intensity and duration of mental work, are some factors which require special attention. The workers even face anxiety when there is no work. The exposure to different environmental conditions like noise, light, heat might be responsible for health impairment (Grandjean, 1998; Latza et al., 2002; Laskar and Murthy, 2004; Maiti, 2008). The women workers at certain point were going through number of job stresses like sexual harassment, jobless, gender based discrimination, proneness to different health hazards, physical problems, insomnia, nausea, headache and other adverse outcome (Chatterji, 2009; Goldenhar et al., 1998; Kakad, 2002; Maiti, 2008; Malenfant et al., 2007; SEWA, 2000). Psychological violence was widespread everywhere, with verbal abuse right at the top followed by bullying and mobbing (Cassitto et al., 2003; De Martino, 2002). Brundtland (2002) reported that health was seriously compromised with causing death of 1.6 million people due to violence and countless more were damaged exposing the many faces of interpersonal, collective and self-directed violence, as well as the settings in which violence occurred. Low support in the workplace increased the rate of absence (Melchior et al., 2003; Niedhammer et al., 1998; North et al., 1996; Vahtera et al., 2000). Abusive supervision was associated with an increase in absenteeism (Tepper et al., 2001). It was found that the workers were highly affected by bullying, mobbing, verbal abuse violence by their seniors or co-workers, leading to moral suppression, depression, frustration, anxiety, followed by absenteeism.

Musculoskeletal Disorder, Accidents and Injuries

Prolonged hours of work in noisy environment, with work burden and psychological stress lead workers to headache. Weight lifting, carrying in awkward position leads to musculoskeletal disorder. This causes back pain, body ache, neck pain, and joint pain. Most of these muscular diseases leads to muscle spasm.

The process of constructing buildings and other structures involves a very wide range of tasks; some of them have certain amount of risks also (Shaun, 2007). This covered various types of occupational diseases, ill health and accident (Gyi et al., 1998; Pritchard, 2004). Dong et al. (1995) observed that working in the construction industry is associated with a high risk of accidents and might result in death in success. A construction project involves a number of small contractors that might lack in terms of technical supervisors and trained workers. They go through traumas like unsafe working condition, falling from height, falling while carrying load etc. This may be resorted to unsafe work practices such as improper building design, lack of guardrails and problems with exits (Shah and Mehta, 2009; TIFAC, 2009; Yuji et al., 2004). Occupational safety hazards in construction might occur due to improper illumination, improper material handling and storage, improper walking and working surfaces, raw concrete surfaces, high platforms, obstructive and unclean floors and aisles, improperly shored trenches and excavations, badly maintained tools, improper scaffoldings, wrongly designed ladders and stairs, unsuitable and badly maintained lifting appliances, unsafe demolition methods, insufficient protection against fire and electric hazards (Andersen and Taylor, 2006; HSE, 2008; Kip Viscusi, 1979). As stated by Decklin (2009), work at height remained the biggest single cause of serious and fatal injuries. Express India (2008) reported that accidental deaths in construction industries is rising at an alarming rate and was considered as the second most hazardous in the world (17%). It is found that in Indian construction industry, the average Fatal Accident Frequency Rate (FAFR) was 15.8 incidents per 1000 employees per year and construction hazards are rated as eight times more risky than those from manufacturing sector (Jain, 2007). The local workers were getting unemployed due to migrant workers who were likely to be the victim of fatal accidents mainly due to non-adherence to adequate safety measures (Chakrabarti, 2008, Rothan, 1985; Safety Media Ltd., 2009). One of the main reasons for high rate of injuries and large number of occupational diseases was low level of occupational health services of the workers (Yu et al., 2002).

Occupational Diseases

Lung diseases like silicosis are also seen among the workers. It is one of the oldest known occupational disease in human being. This happens due to inhalation of dust containing free silica or microscopic crystalline silica beyond its permissible limit. The workers who are exposed to crystalline silica lead to Silicosis, a type of Pneumoconiosis and or cancer (Borm and Donaldson, 1999; Chislom, 1999; Lumen and Spee, 2001; Nij et al., 2002; Nij and Hedrick, 2005). The major occupational diseases in construction industrial workers requiring attention are silicosis, lead poisoning, diseases of joints and bones, carbon monoxide and benzene poising, skin diseases etc. (HSE, 2008; Millon et al., 2007; Oliphant, 1995; Pritchard and Dixon, 2008; TIFAC, 2009).

Difficulty in breathing most probably due to the presence of dust, problem associated with high noise and vibration mostly cause to hearing loss and Raynaud's syndrome respectively (TIFAC, 2009; Thorevskij, 1985). Due to hearing loss the workers speak louder to their colleagues and family members with a concept that others are unable to hear him as he himself could not hear. At working site they do not clean their hands properly. This causes to different types of skin disease affecting their hands and fingers.

Observation

The available literature survey suggested some major problems that the workers are being subjected to. But there is no uniformity and contradictory statements are advocated in some other literatures. It is true that most of the workers are very poor wage earners. They are subjected to different psychosocial stresses resulting in development of health morbidities or diseases. Because of illiteracy, most of the workers state of livelihood was centred on passing the day around with minimum available food and even without any recreational facilities. They even could not think of education for their children. Most of the food consumed are neither supplementing the essential requirements, fat and carbohydrate but lacking even in essential vitamin needs. They are mainly suffering from

- Psychosocial stress
- Job insecurity
- Work burden
- Gender discriminations
- Under nourished
- Back pain
- Joint pain
- Breathlessness
- Severe cough
- Respiratory disease like silicosis

The literature reviewed conveys that out of 60 articles, papers etc., 90 per cent of the workers have low wages and they are poor. They are illiterate. About 35 per cent of the article reveals that they are going through psychosocial stress. This happens due to work burden, monotonous work, job insecurity bullying and mobbing among the workers. Due to psychological stress they are absenting themselves from the work. Around 33.33 per cent of the article reveals that there is risk in the work and they go through accident and injuries while at work. It was found that 25 per cent of the articles were about the respiratory ailments or diseases. Some skin diseases were there in most of the workers due to exposure to the work. Around 16.67 per cent of the papers reveal that the workers were aware of different social security measures.

Conclusion

The workers are required to be educated. They must use social security measures like masks, gloves, helmets while at work. This will help them in prevention of risk factors which they assess while at work. Government of India has promulgated different Acts and rules for the building construction workers. To safeguard their health different social security schemes are available. It is required to make the worker aware by individual counselling. Necessity for seeking medical attention is also required. Studies are required from different disciplines for their upliftment from all aspects of their life.

References

Andersen, M.L. and H.F. Taylor. 2006. *Sociology: Understanding a Diverse Society*. Thomson Wadsworth, Belmont CA.

Borm, P.J.A. and K. Donaldson. 1999. The Quartz Hazard in Construction Industry. *Indoor and Built Environment,* 8: 107–12.

Brundtland, G.H. 2002. Preface, in E.G. Krug , L.L. Dahlberg, J. A. Mercy , A. B. Zwi , R. Lozano (eds.) *World Report on Violence and Health.* World Health Organization, Geneva.

Cassitto, M.G., E. Fattorini, R. Gilioli, C. Rengo, and V. Gonik. 2003. *Raising Awareness of Psychological Harassment at Work.* World Health Organization, Geneva.

Census of India. 2001. Economic Activity; *NIC Classification; West Bengal.* Ministry of Home Affairs, Government of India.

Chakrabarti, D. 2005. *India Construction Industry and Workers.* Construction Workers Federation of India, Kolkata.

——. 2008. *Globalisation and Migrant Labour.* Construction Workers Federation of India, Kolkata.

Chatterji, S.A. 2009. Women and Work in the Informal Sector. *The Sunday Statesman,* 14 June, p. 7.

Chishlom, J. 1999. Respirable Dust and Respirable Silica Concentration from Construction Activities. *Indoor and Built Environment.* 8 (2): 94–106.

Cox, T., M. Thirlaway, C. Watts, S. Cox, and C. Mackay. 1979. Job Stress: The Effects of Repetitive Work. Department of Employment Gazette (London, 1: 234–37.

Das, S. 2007. Workers in Unorganised Sector Lack Social Security. *Down to Earth,* 30 June.

Decklin, B. 2009. *Construction Accident Claims.* <http://www.articles zone.com/articledirectory>. 11 February 2011.

Di Martino V. 2002. *Workplace Violence in the Health Sector: Country Case Studies Brazil, Bulgaria, Lebanon, Portugal, South Africa, Thailand Plus an Additional Australian Study:* Synthesis Report, ILO/ICN/WHO/ PSI Joint Programme on Workplace Violence in the Health Sector, Geneva.

Dong, W., P. Vaughan, K. Sullivan, and T. Fletcher. 1995. Mortality Study of Construction Workers in the UK. *International Journal of Epidemiology,* 24 (4): 750–57.

Express India. 2008. 28 April Is Construction Worker Memorial Day. *Express News Service,* 28 April .

Fernandez, D. and G.D. Bino Paul. 2011. Social Networks of Migrant Construction Workers in Goa, *The Indian Journal of Industrial Relations,* 47 (1): 65–77.

Goldenhar, L.M., N.G. Swanson, J.J. Hurrell Jr, A. Ruder, and J. Deddens. 1998. Stressors and Adverse Outcomes for Female Construction Workers. *J Occu Health Psychol,* 3 (1): 19–32.

Grandjean, E. 1998. Fatigue, in *Encyclopaedia of Occupational Health and Safety I.* ILO Geneva, pp: 837–39.

Gyi, D.E., R.A. Haslam and A.G.F. Gibb. 1998. Case Studies of Occupational Health Management in the Engineering Construction Industry. *Occupational Medicine,* 48: 263–71.

Health and Safety Executive. 2008. Managing Occupational Health Risks in Construction. www.hse.gov.uk/construction/healthrisk/ index.htm. 11 February 2011.

Jain, S.K. 2007. *Meeting the Challenges in Industrial Safety Management in Construction Industry*. Nuclear Power Corporation of India Ltd, Mumbai.

Kakad, K. 2002. Gender Discrimination in the Construction Industry: The Case of Two Cities in India. *Gender, Technology and Development*, 6 (3): 355–72.

Kip Viscusi, W. 1979. *Employment Hazards: An Investigation of Market Performance*. Harvard University Press, Cambridge.

Lakhani, R. 2004. Occupational Health of Women Construction Workers in the Unorganised Sector. *Journal of Health Management*, 6 (2): 187–200.

Laskar, A. and C.V.R. Murthy. 2004. *Challenges before Construction Industry in India*, Indian Institute of Technology, Kanpur.

Latza, U., A. Pfahlberg and O. Gefeller. 2002. Impact of Repetitive Manual Materials Handling and Psychosocial Work Factors on the Future Prevalence of Chronic Low-back Pain among Construction Workers. *Scand J Work Environ Health*, 28 (5): 314–23.

Lumens, M.E.G.L. and T. Spee. 2001. Determinants of Exposure to Respirable Quartz Dust in the Construction Industry. *Ann. Occup. Hyg*, 45 (7): 585–95.

Maiti, R. 2008. Workload Assessment in Building Construction Related Activities in India. *Applied Ergonomics*, 39 (6): 754–65.

Malenfant, R., A. La Rue and M. Vezina. 2007. Intermittent Work and Well-being. *Current Sociology*, 55 (6): 814–35.

Melchior, M., I. Niedhammer, L.F. Berkman, and M. Goldberg. 2003. Do Psychosocial Work Factors and Social Relations Exert Independent Effects on Sickness Absence? A Six Year Prospective Study of the GAZEL Cohort. *Journal of Epidemiology and Community Health*, 57: 285–93.

Milon, Antoine, Sottas Pierre-Edouard, Bulliard Jean-Luc, and Vernez David. 2007. Effective Exposure to Solar UV in Building Workers: Influence of Local and Individual Factors. *Journal of Exposure Science & Environmental Epidemiology*, 17 (1): 58–68.

Ministry of Planning, Government of India. 1987. *Revised National Industrial Classification of all Economic Activities* (NIC). CSO, Department of Statistics. 7.

Ministry of Labour and Employment, Government of India. 1996. *Building and Other Construction Workers (Regulation of Employment and Working Conditions) Act, 1996*. Government of India, New Delhi.

National Commission for Enterprises in the Unorganised Sector (NCEUS). 2006. Report on Social Security for Unorganised Workers, NCEUS. Government of India, New Delhi.

National Sample Survey Organisation (NSSO). 2008. *Employment and Unemployment Situation in India 2005–06, NSS 62nd Round,* Ministry of Statistics and Programme Implementation, Government of India.

Niedhammer, I., I. Bugel, M. Goldberg, A. Leclerc, and A. Gueguen. 1998. Psychosocial Factors at Work and Sickness Absence in the Gazel Cohort: A Prospective Study. *Occupational and Environmental Medicine,* 55: 735–41.

Nij, E.T. and D. Hedrick. 2005. Risk Assessment of Silicosis and Lung Cancer Among Construction Workers Exposed to Resipirable Quartz. *Scand J. Work Environ. Health,* 31 (2): 49–56.

Nij, E.T., P. Borm, D. Höhr, and D. Heederik. 2002. Pneumoconiosis and Exposure to Quartz-Containing Dust in the Construction Industry. *Ann. Occup. Hyg,* 46 (1): 71–76.

North, F.M., S.L. Syme, A. Feeney, M. Shipley, and M. Marmot. 1996. Psychosocial Work Environment and Sickness Absence among British Civil Servants: The Whitehall II Study. *American Journal of Public Health,* 86: 332–40.

Oliphant, J. 1995. Taking Account of the Occupational Hazards. *Construction news.* < http://www.cnplus.co.uk>. 11 February 2011.

Paycheck India. 2009. Minimum Wages India: Current Minimum Wage Rate India. IIM, Ahmedabad, <www.paycheckindia.com>. 11 February 2011.

Pritchard, C. 2004. Building for Health? The Construction Managers of Tomorrow. *The Journal of Royal Society for the Promotion of Health,* 124 (4): 171–76.

Pritchard, C. and P.B. Dixon. 2008. Reporting of Skin Cancer Risks in the House-building Industry: Alternative Approaches to the Analysis of Categorical Data. *Public Health,* 122 (3): 237–42.

Rajasekhar, D., J.Y. Suchitra, S. Madheswaran, and G.K. Karanath. 2009. At Times When Limbs May Fail: Social Security for Unorganised Workers in Karnataka. *Karmayaoga,* 1–32.

Rajawat, M. 2003. Schedule Castes in India. *History,* 218.

Ramesh, P.B. 2009. Rethinking Social Protection for India's Working Poor in the Unorganised Sector, *Cross National Policy Exchange: Asia Social Protection Papers,* 1–18.

Rothan, A. 1985. Migrant Workers, in *Encyclopaedia of Occupational Health and Safety II*: International Labour Organization, Geneva, 1359–61.

Safety Media Ltd. 2009. Migrant Construction Workers 'more at risk'. < http://www.safetymedia.co.uk/>.

Sarkar, P. 2008. *Working Hours of Adults, Factories Act, 1948 with Short Notes*. Book N Books Publishers and Booksellers, Kolkata.

SEWA Academy. 2000. *Labouring Brick by Brick: A Study on Construction Workers*. Self Employed Women's Association (SEWA), Ahmedabad.

Shah, C.K. and H. Mehta. 2009. Study of Injuries among Construction Workers in Ahmedabad City, Gujarat. *Indian Journal for the Practicing Doctors*, 5: 6.

Shaun, A. 2007. Health and Safety Accidents and the Causes Analysis within the Construction Industry. *Aberdeen University Press Services*, 1–56.

Snashall, D. 2007. Preventing Occupational Illhealth in the Construction Industry. *Occupational and Environmental Medicine*, 64: 789–90.

Tepper, B. J., M.K. Duffy and J.D. Shaw. 2001. Personality Moderators of the Relationship between Abusive Supervision and Subordinates' Resistance. *Journal of Applied Psychology*, 86: 974–83.

Thorevskij, V.I. 1985. Monotonous Work, in *Encyclopaedia of Occupational Health and Safety-II*. International Labour Organization , Geneva, 1405–6.

TIFAC. 2009. *Technology Information, Forecasting and Assessment Council*, Industrial Safety and Hazard Management in Construction Industry, Department of Science and Technology, Government of India.

Vahtera, J., M. Kivimäki, J. Pentti, and T. Theorell. 2000. Effect of Change in the Psychosocial Work Environment on Sickness Absence: A Seven Year Follow up of Initially Healthy Employees. *Journal of Epidemiology and Community Health*, 54: 484–93.

Yu, T.S.I., F.F.K. Cheng, S.L.A. Tse, and T. Wong W. 2002. Assessing the Provision of Occupational Health Services in the Construction Industry in Hong Kong, *Occupational Medicine*, 52: 375–82.

Yuji, N., H. Toshio, S. Mari, and T. Naoki. 2004. Asbestos-related Diseases among Construction Workers in Japan. *Asian-Pacific Newsletter*, 11 (1): 10–14.

CHAPTER 7

Socio-Economic Impact on Health

A Study of the Cycle Rikshaw Wallas of Kolkata

SOVAN CHAKRABORTY

Health and well-being is a much larger domain, which affects all aspects of human existence. It has a wider implication for social, economic and political life of an individual and indeed cannot be fully understood within the sphere of medical models. Somehow, it is very difficult to define a person having 'good health' but it is certainly more than just the absence of diseases. Health reflects a state of mental, social and physical fitness and well-being of the individual and it is strongly influenced by his or her lifestyle (Dash Sharma, 2004). Health is man's natural condition. It is the result of living in accordance with natural laws pertaining to the body, mind and environment. These laws relate to fresh air, sunlight, exercise, rest and relaxation, sleep, cleanliness, elimination, right attitude of mind, good habits and above all lifestyle (Sachchidananda, 1994). Health is now recognised as a birth right of all citizens. With the adoption of health as an integral part of socio-economic development by the United Nations in 1979, health while being an end in itself has also become a major instrument of overall socio-economic development and the criterion of a new social order (UNDP, 2003). World Health Organization has defined 'Health as a state of complete physical, mental and social well being and not merely an absence of disease or infirmity' (WHO, 1948).

In India, the term informal sector has not been used in the official statistics or in the National Accounts Statistics (NAS). The terms in the Indian NAS are 'Organized and Unorganized' sectors. The National Sample Survey Organization (NSSO) carried out a sample survey in 1999–2000 and its results showed that out of total workforce of 397 million, only 28 million workers are employed in the organised sector and remaining in the unorganised sector (NSSO, 2001).

Cycle rickshaws are known as *cyclo* (pronounced see-clo) in Cambodia and Vietnam, *cycle rickshaw* in India and Bangladesh, *samlor* (literally 'three wheels') in Thailand, *trishaw* from 'tricycle rickshaws' in Malaysia and Singapore, and *becak* in Indonesia. The first rickshaws appeared in Japan around 1868, with the beginning of the Meiji period. Around 1880, rickshaws appeared in India, first in Simla and then, 20 years later, in Calcutta (Ganguly, 1982). Here they were initially used by Chinese traders to transport goods; in 1914 the Chinese applied for permission to use rickshaws to transport passengers. Soon after, rickshaws appeared in many big cities in Southeast Asia; pulling and pedalling a rickshaw was often the first job for peasants migrating to these cities. According to estimates in the Indian Transportation context, cycle rickshaws are plying over 7 million passengers or goods in various Indian cities and towns including 20 States and Union Territories (Sinha, 2008). Cycle rickshaws meet mobility requirements of urban dwellers in low and middle income areas and tourist places of numerous cities. It also provides low-cost alternative for carrying short distance passengers, household goods and construction and business materials. Cycle rickshaw *wallas* are the most important category of the informal sector in the urban situation, as they live at one corner of the society. The growing informal sectors in the mega cities in India have provided economic opportunities to the immigrant population (Warren, 1994). Owing to disparity in economic development among different regions, people from one region to the other migrate towards the metropolitan centre. City becomes a place for assimilation of different culture (Michael, 1989). They each tend to be ostracised and so suffer various forms of social exclusion. Cycle rickshaw wallas spend a sizeable amount of their incomes to mitigate health shocks, indicating for them a high level of health vulnerability (Tauhidul, 1995). But there are a number of socio-economic factors which are a great hindrance for health and these are creating a number of health hazards to the people. This particular condition was studied in the present studies among cycle rickshaw wallas in ward no 92 of Dhakuria, South Kolkata.

Objectives

The purpose of this study, firstly, is to identify the cycle rickshaw wallas migration and socio-economic condition. Secondly, to study the general health status of the studied people and to identify the major influencing factors responsible for health. The last one is to observe how socio-economic conditions responsible for their health status.

Methods of Study

The work included the broad themes of collecting data like observation of the area basically the cycle rickshaw stands and cycle rickshaw wallas' socio-economic life. The study is based on a sample of cycle rickshaw wallas, who at the time of a survey, were living and pursuing their economic activity in Dhakuria, South Kolkata. All cycle rickshaw wallas were interviewed using more detailed structured schedules and case studies. For case studies the informants were selected by purposive selection. Through the case study method the condition of cycle rickshaw wallas have been very conspicuous to us. It has revealed their pain, sorrow and desire for education of their children who are missed at the time of lunch by their father. Data have also been collected through interview schedules. Apart from this, personal observation was helpful to obtain more serious living condition and their homes in squatter settlements.

Studied Area and the People

The present fieldwork was conducted among the cycle rickshaw wallas of Dhakuria at ward number 92 in the South Kolkata. In South Kolkata, Dhakuria is a big area connected by both trains and buses. The Gariahat road (South), which passes over Dhakuria bridge and bus stand as well as Southern railway which passes over Dhakuria, are very important for communication. Many schools and hospitals are located in and around Dhakuria. The train runs parallel to Dhakuria and bus plies on the main road to different directions of South to North of Kolkata and suburbs. Many narrow roads, lanes and bye lanes connect different hamlets of Dhakuria, which are only accessible by cycle rickshaws. Cycle rickshaws provide cheap, reliable and consumer friendly transport options in a city where the buses are irredeemably dirty, crowded and dangerous and the car and taxis are unaffordable for the majority of the citizens. They are particularly useful for women, the elderly, the frail, and the disabled. The cycle rickshaw wallas take customers at any hour of the day or night, will work during the worst of the monsoons and through the more waterlogged streets and will take children to and from school in a city where personal care and reliability are highly valued. This study has been conducted at 10 cycle rickshaw stands and among 200 cycle rickshaw wallas.

Effects of Migration

Migration plays a vital role in social life of any community to change the status of the people. Migration is the movement of population from one place to another. Migration has been a common phenomenon in Indian subcontinent. The studied people were residing mainly in and around Kolkata mainly in slum areas and in *dera* or rented rooms sharing 2 to 3 rickshaw wallas. Among the studied 200 families, 145 families were migrants and 55 were non-migrants. The non-migrant people were residing mainly in Kolkata especially in Dhakuria and its surrounding areas, i.e., both 24 Parganas. The migration of the studied population had started after independence and it is still going on. Among the migrant families 103 (51.50%) families came from different districts of West Bengal, 32 (16.00%) families were from different states of India and 10 (5.00%) families came from outside India, i.e., Bangladesh (Table 1). The oldest cases of migration took place in the 1950s or after independence and the latest took place in the year 2004. The highest numbers of migration were noticed during 1960–69 and 1970–79 mainly for war and several political reason. The migration from Bangladesh took place during that time. Large numbers of families were coming from Bihar, Jharkhand and Orissa to West Bengal mainly for search of new occupation. Migration took place from these areas in and around Kolkata because the people had lost their previous occupation due to war, natural calamities and different other reasons. So, migration from villages to the cities depends on various factors, most important of which is economic factor. Expanding employment opportunities in the cities attract people from surrounding areas. Kolkata is a place where people come for better employment opportunities. This is the place where people come from different states of India and engage themselves in different activities.

Table 1

Migration of Rickshaw Wallas

Types	*No of Families*	*%*
Non-Migrant	55	27.50
Within West Bengal	103	51.50
Outside West Bengal	32	16.00
Outside India-Bangladesh	10	5.00
Total	200	100.00

Age of Entry and Period of Involvement to the Profession

Age is a vital factor in this profession. It was found that the cycle rickshaw wallas vary in terms of age. Some rickshaw wallas are older in age and others are young. In any profession age is a matter of concern, but here age is a bar. If a person is old he will not be carrying enough loads. Children of below 15 years and old persons are not generally encouraged because there is risk of accident while carrying passenger. Table 2 and 3 shows the age of entry into this profession and age group wise distribution and period of involvement in this job. Table 2 depicts that total 13.50 per cent rickshaw wallas started to pedal rickshaw when their age was 15–19 years. Total 31.00 per cent rickshaw wallas started their rickshaw pedalling at the age of 20–24 years. Total 37.50 per cent rickshaw wallas started this profession at the age of 25–29 years. Total 13.50 per cent rickshaw wallas started to pedal rickshaw at the age of 30–34 years. Total 4.50 per cent rickshaw started to pedal rickshaw at the age of 35–39 years. It is clear that no rickshaw wallas below 15 years and above 40 years of age were found pedalling rickshaw.

Table 2

Age of Entry to this Profession

Age (in Years)	*No. of Rickshaw Wallas*	*%*
15–19	27	13.50
20–24	62	31.00
25–29	75	37.50
30–34	27	13.50
35–39	9	4.50
Total	200	100.00

Table 3

Age Group wise Distribution and Period of Involvement in this Job

Age Groups (in Years)	*No of Cycle Rickshaw Wallas*	*%*	*Period of Involvement in this Job*				
			Below 5 Years	*5–10 Years*	*10–15 Years*	*15–20 Years*	*20+ Years*
Below 20	3	1.5	3	—	—	—	—
20–24	12	6	10	2	—	—	—
25–29	59	29.5	35	18	6	—	—
30–34	47	23.5	7	28	12	—	—
35–39	33	16.5	—	13	11	9	—
40–44	21	10.5	1	7	8	4	1
45–49	11	5.5	—	1	4	3	3
50–54	7	3.5	—	—	—	2	5
55–59	5	2.5	—	—	—	2	3
60–64	2	1	—	—	—	1	1
Total	200	100	56 (28.00%)	69 (34.50%)	41 (20.50%)	21 (10.50%)	13 (6.50%)

The Table 3 shows the age group wise distribution of cycle rickshaw wallas. Here total 29.50 per cent and 23.50 per cent rickshaw wallas belong to the age group of 25–29 and 30–34 years respectively. Total 16.50 per cent and 10.50 per cent rickshaw wallas fall in the age group between 35–39 years and 40–44 years respectively. In the age group between 45–49 years the percentage of rickshaw wallas is 5.50 per cent. Total 3.50 per cent and 2.50 per cent rickshaw wallas are present in the age group between 50–54 years and 55–59 years respectively. In the age group between 60–64 years the percentage of rickshaw wallas is 1 per cent. So, rickshaw wallas below 25 years old are not present in this table. There was no rickshaw walla above 64 years. The numbers of rickshaw wallas decrease as the age group increase.

It was found that many cycle rickshaw wallas were involved in this job since long years. Some of them were involved since 20–25 years in this job. Some were newcomers in the profession. So, period of involvement is another factor that reflects their socio-economic life around this profession. As compared with those people who were old in this profession and those who were newcomers, a slight difference was observed in their social and economic life. Both the groups lead a simple life and their socio-economic conditions were very poor. Total 6.50 per cent people were working in this occupation since more than 20 years, 10.50 per cent were engaged in this job since 15–20 years ago. The Table 3 shows that the numbers of rickshaw wallas below 20 years were three and above 55 years were five. With the increasing age, the number of people decrease due to their age and poor health.

Entry to the New Occupation

The rickshaw stand is not open for all. Each stand has a limited number of rickshaw capacities. So, taking entry to the stand is very important. It is important to know how they had entry to the stand. Each stand has its own procedure to join as new cycle rickshaw wallas. New cycle rickshaw wallas had to pay a certain amount of money to the stand committee. When an old cycle rickshaw wallas leave any stand and in a case of death of someone then the new comers who have paid money to the committee are registered as permanent rickshaw wallas of the stand. Table 4 shows that how the rickshaw wallas came to this profession from their previous occupation.

Table 4

Previous Occupations of Rickshaw Wallas

Previous Occupation	*No and Percentage of Rickshaw Wallas*	*%*
As an Agricultural Labourer	105	52.50
Day Labourer	52	26.00
Small Businessman	4	2.00
As a Rickshaw Puller	27	13.50
Work in Hotel as Cook	12	6.00
Total	200	100.00

Previous occupations of the studied people were mainly as agricultural labourer and day labourer, few were small businessmen, cooks and rickshaw pullers. But their income was very low. So, they are moved to city in search of better occupation and they chose rickshaw pedalling in the urban area which improved their situation little bit. Another reason of their coming in city was that agriculture is done for a certain time of year but not throughout whereas rickshaw pedalling is done every time of the year.

Economic Condition

Income of cycle rickshaw wallas is dependent on their period of involvement in this job. If a cycle rickshaw walla works more than 12 hours he earns more. But other person who pedals rickshaw only for 6 to 7 hours earns less. Other factor is age group. The older people do not work more than 10 hours but younger people work more. So, their income level is high. Those rickshaw wallas have some subsidiary occupation, they have some extra income. But, when they did other work, they ignored rickshaw pedalling. So, it affects their income level too. Considering the family income 29 cycle rickshaw wallas could earn below ₹ 2000 per month (14.50%), 104 (52.00%) rickshaw wallas earn between ₹ 2001–3500 per month, 51 (25.50%) rickshaw wallas earn between ₹ 3501–5000 per month and only 16 (8.00%) rickshaw wallas had the monthly income more than ₹ 5001. Their average family member was five in number and with this mere source of income it would be rather very hard for them to fulfill the daily livelihood requirement of the family members.

Table 5

Income of Rickshaw Wallas

Per Month Income of Rickshaw Wallas	*No of Rickshaw Wallas*	*%*
Below 2000	29	14.50
₹ 2001–3500	104	52.00
₹ 3501–5000	51	25.50
More than ₹ 5001	16	8.00
Total	200	100.00

Ownership of Rickshaws

Some of the cycle rickshaw wallas were owner of their own cycle rickshaws, but others hired cycle rickshaw from those persons who had more than one cycle rickshaw. The owner of cycle rickshaw generally makes a contract with non-owner. The non-owner paid rupees 15 per day or ₹ 300 per month, to the owner of cycle rickshaw.

Maintenance of the Rickshaw

Maintenance of rickshaws is very important. Among the studied cycle rickshaw stands, no new rickshaws are found, all rickshaws are older and the conditions of the rickshaws are not good. Some of them are very hard and not so old but others are in poor condition and old. The owner rickshaw wallas maintain their own rickshaws. But those who rent the rickshaws has a mutual contract with the owner. The contract is, when the cycle rickshaws are heavily damaged like tyre burst, damage in mudguard, ring, spoke, chain etc. the owners repair their own cycle rickshaws. But in case of small damage like leaks, pumping etc. it is done by the renter. In every month some rupees are expended behind cycle rickshaws for maintenance. At times expenditure is huge but normally it is small in amount based on damaging condition of the cycle rickshaws.

Time of Cycle Rickshaw Pedalling

Rickshaw walla's source of income is based on rickshaw pedalling. If one rickshaw walla works 6.00 A.M. to 10.00 P.M. per day he earns more than ₹200. But this is not possible for older and aged cycle rickshaw wallas. Not all but some middle aged and young rickshaw wallas have worked between 6.00 A.M. to 9 P.M. Working time is a vital factor for all cycle rickshaw wallas. Another important factor is pick hours of the stand when passengers come regularly. This factor is varying from one stand to another. So, time is related to cycle rickshaw wallas per day income. In every stand cycle rickshaw pedalling started at 6.00

A.M. and continued till 10.00 P.M. All rickshaw wallas are not pedalling the rickshaw from 6.00 A.M. to 10.00 P.M. Some cycle rickshaw wallas pedal rickshaw in morning, some in the afternoon and some in the evening. In summer time the aged rickshaw wallas pedal rickshaw in morning time because of temperature.

Educational Scenario

Education is the basic requirement for getting a good job. But in this kind of profession education is not required. Without education one can join this occupation. Table 6 show the educational level of the cycle rickshaw wallas has been shown. Total 30.50 per cent cycle rickshaw wallas are illiterate and 69.30 per cent literate. Among literate 17.00 per cent rickshaw wallas can only sign. Rickshaw wallas who have studied up to class IV is 28 per cent and 11 per cent rickshaw wallas have studied up to class VIII. Only 4 per cent are in class IX and X and 2.50 per cent rickshaw wallas have been in the higher secondary level and above. All rickshaw wallas come from poorer family. Some rickshaw wallas' father died at an early age. So entire family pressure was fallen upon him and due to absence of any guidance they joined the gang of bad boys and started smoking and drinking etc. It has been found that the uneducated rickshaw wallas admire the educated one and take necessary help from them regarding legal and money matters. The general trend shows that rickshaw pedalling is associated with lower educational level. This is the profession where most of the people had to leave school for some economic problem and when they required a job, they did not get better opportunity than this. This affects to the next generation; they could not give care and attention at all over the studies of their children. Due to their economic constraints it would be rather impossible for the concerned families to provide higher education to their children. Educational dropout was a very common feature specially in the higher school level.

Table 6

Educational Level of Rickshaw Wallas

Types	*No*	*%*
Illiterate	61	30.50
Can sign only	34	17.00
Below Primary	13	6.50
Class I–IV	56	28.00
Class V–VIII	23	11.50
Class IX–X	8	4.00
Higher Secondary and above	5	2.50
Total	200	100.00

House Types and Settlement Patterns

The poor level of income provides a very little chance to acquire better livelihood conditions. Most of the families reside in a single room. Positions of kitchen were mostly inside rooms but in few cases they cooked outside rooms. Most of the houses devoid proper drainage and sanitary system and for this purpose they used the common bathroom and common tap and tubewell water. In the context of health and hygiene the surrounding environment of the houses were mostly poor in condition. Due to improper drainage system water storage was seen all the time of the year and in rainy seasons the situation is very bad and it became the key birth place of various germs. Most (51.50%) rickshaw wallas lived in rented house in Dhakuria and its surrounding areas with their families (Table 7). Total 30.50 per cent rickshaw wallas lived in their own houses with their families but 18.00 per cent lived in *Dera* individually. *Dera* is nothing but a rented room in urban area like Dhakuria, which is rented by two or more rickshaw wallas individually. Their family stays in villages and rural areas.

Table 7

Types of Houses

Type of Houses	*In Dera*	*In Rented House*	*In their Own House*
Percentage of Rickshaw Wallas	36 (18.00%)	103 (51.50%)	61 (30.50%)

Socio-Economic Factors Affecting Health

Effects of migration results the rickshaw wallas leave their early occupational pattern as well as early settlements. In earlier occupation majority of them engaged in agricultural sector. As a result the previous surrounding environmental background was changed and they were exposed in a new ecological niche. Their new settlements and new occupation provide them a new way of living. Generally the new environmental scenario brought new cultural practices to them. They were working throughout the day and in any seasons, i.e., warm summer, extreme cold and excessive rain. The rickshaw's are non-polluting but the working atmosphere is a dusty and polluted one. Naturally, the working atmosphere brings a number of health hazards to them.

The little amount of income was a severe constraint for the poor families to consume the adequate balance diet. Foods are related to economy. In higher economic status people take good, better quality and expensive food. But people under poverty line do not take expensive and better quality food. Cycle rickshaw walla's daily foods are based on their economic condition. Most of them eat *panta* (cold rice with water) in the morning. Some of them eat bread and curry, others eat *chattu*. In afternoon they take lunch from hotel. But who stay near or at Dhakuria eat in their home. But the rickshaw wallas who come from Garia, Sonarpur and outside Dhakuria, eat lunch in hotels. In the evening most rickshaw wallas take tea and tiffin. Their tiffin includes mainly puffed rice, bread, *ghugni*, etc. from tea stall near Dhakuria bus and rail station. At night they eat in their home. They mainly eat rice. I did not find any person who ate bread at night. All people ate boiled rice with curry at night. Majority of cycle rickshaw wallas drink country liquor or *cholai* everyday. Some of them drink *cholai* occasionally. Everyone smokes *biri*, some of them eat *pan, taranga, shaker, gutka* etc.

Drinking water and water usage of household work gives another highlighting issue. More than 65 per cent of the families were depended on the tap water of the municipalities and 45 per cent were depended on tubewell for the said purpose. They consume water without any sort of disinfection and boiling which may result in serious water borne diseases like dysentery.

This occupation itself results a number of health hazards to the studied people. They spend a sizeable amount of their income to mitigate health shocks, indicating for them a high level of health vulnerability. This section deals with the health status, disease and health cure treatment of rickshaw wallas. The data about health and disease were collected at the time of survey during last one year from all the rickshaw wallas. The Tables 8 and 9 shows the name of disease and number of affected cycle rickshaw wallas as well as the nature of treatment.

Table 8

Name of Disease and No. of Affected Cycle Rickshaw Wallas (During last one year at the time of study)

Name of the Disease	*No of Affected Cases*	*Percentage against the 200 Rickshaw Wallas*
Arthritis	1	0.50
Anemia	9	4.50
Asthma	6	3.00
Cough and Cold	25	12.50
Chicken Pox	4	2.00
Diarrhoea	17	8.50
Dysentery	23	11.50
Eye Problem	7	3.50
Fever	35	17.50
Jaundice	16	8.00
Malaria	31	15.50
Mumps	2	1.00
Physical Injury Due to Accident	14	7.00
Respiratory Problem and Chest Pain	39	19.50
Skin Diseases	4	2.00
Stomach Upset and Abdominal Pain	21	10.50
Tuberculosis	3	1.50
Typhoid	8	4.00
No. of Cases	265	—

Table 9

Number of Disease Affected Person and Nature of Treatment

Name of the Diseases	*Allopathic*	*%*	*Homeo-pathy*	*%*	*Quack*	*%*	*Tradi-tional*	*%*
Arthritis	1	0.38	0	0.00	0	0.00	0	0.00
Anemia	3	1.13	4	1.51	0	0.00	2	0.75
Asthma	1	0.38	5	1.89	0	0.00	0	0.00
Cough and Cold	5	1.89	2	0.75	15	5.66	3	1.13
Chicken Pox	0	0.00	0	0.00	1	0.38	3	1.13
Diarrhoea	7	2.64	0	0.00	10	3.77	0	0.00
Dysentery	8	3.02	6	2.26	7	2.64	2	0.75
Eye Problem	2	0.75	1	0.38	4	1.51	0	0.00
Fever	11	4.15	4	1.51	15	5.66	5	1.89
Jaundice	2	0.75	4	1.51	2	0.75	8	3.02
Malaria	8	3.02	5	1.89	15	5.66	3	1.13
Mumps	0	0.00	1	0.38	1	0.38	0	0.00
Physical Injury Due to Accident	12	4.53	0	0.00	2	0.75	0	0.00
Respiratory Problem and Chest Pain	9	3.40	12	4.53	10	3.77	8	3.02
Skin Diseases	0	0.00	3	1.13	0	0.00	1	0.38
Stomach Upset and Abdominal Pain	9	3.40	4	1.51	6	2.26	2	0.75
Tuberculosis	1	0.38	0	0.00	2	0.75	0	0.00
Typhoid	5	1.89	1	0.38	2	0.75	0	0.00
Total	84	31.70	52	19.62	92	34.72	37	13.96

At the time of survey total 265 cases of types of disease affected by rickshaw wallas were recorded. But all the cases were not critical or serious disease, few were short term disease also. Short term disease like fever, cough with cold, head and eye injury from accidents, dysentery and stomach upset etc., Total 18 numbers of diseases were recorded from the Table 8. Short term diseases were seen often among them and they got partial recovery from them with a little treatment. But other diseases which they suffered was from long period and it required proper medical check up. But often negligence over short term diseases made them complex ones and it had turned out as a serious problem to them. Their continuous work in the dusty and polluted road as well as carbon and carbon monoxide emitted from the buses and the cars, repeatedly being inhaled by them through their respiration might have caused acute respiratory problem and chest pain which may turn into chronic asthma. Lack of proper nutritive food and hard manual labour may had resulted acute nutritional imbalance among them and it had turned into anaemia. From field survey it was noticed that lack of proper nutrition, heavy work load together with polluted environment and their alcoholism as well as smoking may have resulted this disease.

Most of the people with their ailments went to the charitable medical centre and health centre for primary treatment but it was not always providing with adequate medicines and necessary diagnostic tests. The Table 9 discussed about the treatment method of the studied people. The concerned people with numerous suffering went to government hospitals for treatment. But they were unable to bear expenses regarding medicines and other required clinical diagnostic. They could not seek medical consultancy from the private doctors or nursing home. To get treatment from diseases they first of all went to the quack doctors and the local medical shops because the medicine provided by the quacks gave them a quick remedy and they could rejoin their work. Besides this they have strong belief on traditional method specially on evil spirits and evil eye. According to them those evil eye and spirits creates a number of physical and mental problem to the affected persons. They also were going to the magico-religious healers and local *Kabiraj*. They had a psychological faith on them that they could prevent the effect of evil spirits rather than modern medical practices. Another reason for them to go to the traditional medicine practitioners was because of high price of modern medicines and high fees of modern medical practices. To cure the patients those traditional healers provided them sanctified lockets, *tel pora, jolpora,* and traditional medicine from medicinal plants. Their busy working schedule and lack of educational awareness were a root cause behind it.

So, among all cycle rickshaw wallas, acute health problem arises primarily from cold and fever, gastroenteric problem including acidity and pains and physical weakness. Chronic illness of the rickshaw wallas are also linked primarily to gastroenteric problems, aches and pain. Hence, a significant part of the health vulnerability of the rickshaw wallas may be classified as occupational hazards. Injuries accounted by accidents was a major illness of rickshaw wallas. According to the perceptions of illness and of the major health hazards are directly or indirectly connected to rickshaw pedalling itself. While some road accidents and injuries are straight forward examples, other possible job-related hazards pointed out by the cycle rickshaw wallas are eating unhygienic food from roadside stalls, hotels and eating irregularly rickshaw pedalling in adverse weather conditions like scorching heat or incessant rains and of course physical exhaustion.

General Observations

Cycle rickshaws provide cheap, reliable and consumer friendly transport options in Kolkata. The cycle rickshaws of Kolkata are non-polluting. It provides desperately needed employment for citizens on the knife edge of existence and they support many hundreds and thousands of dependents both in Kolkata and home areas of those migrant workers who feel the jobs of cycle rickshaw wallas. This profession requires less skill, less education and it does not require ample investment, too. These people depend on their labour mostly to earn their livelihood. Rickshaw pedalling is their personal achievement to solve some unemployment problem at the present time.

Urban cycle rickshaw wallas come from a very poor economic background consistent with the characteristics of chronic poverty. Rickshaw pedalling provides a route of modest upward mobility for those among the rural chronic poor who come to the city for work. The rickshaw wallas are susceptible to systematic health risks. Deteriorating health combined with health shocks can impose a significant burden on the urban poor rickshaw wallas, dragging down the pace of upward mobility during their lifetime. The activity of rickshaw pedalling represents an unsustainable livelihood, as the initial welfare gain tapers off with length of involvement in the sector. Intergenerational mobility of rickshaw wallas households is constrained by very limited schooling and the poor range of occupational choices for children. Moreover, this profession is provided to poor young people who find new ways and new opportunities for themselves in urban economic sector. Some countries and cities have banned or restricted cycle rickshaws. They are often prohibited in congested areas of major cities.

The present health situation of the rickshaw wallas is not a result of a day or two but the concerned fact lies in an earlier situation and it is totally related with their socio-economic condition. Due to migration the rickshaw wallas had lost their traditional occupation and they also leave their traditional homeland. In a new environmental condition they started a new way of life with new occupation. Their new occupation provides them more money than their previous occupation but due to huge expenditure in urban areas they were suffering from acute financial crisis. For that reasons they had prevented them to acquire nutritious diet required for their heavy work load. On the other hand they have limited educational awareness. Under this circumstances the knowledge regarding health and hygienic was suffering a major set back. These factors were not at all preventing their diseases but rather it makes their suffering more aggravated. With the changing environment a lot of cultural practices had changed among them. They had a general consensus to go to the traditional healers and common faith on them regarding health care practices. In urban areas the number of traditional health care system and the traditional healers were less in number. For the cure of diseases they had to go to the rural areas. It was too much costlier among them. But the traditional healers were unable to fulfill all their demand in most of the cases. So the people were not only depended on healers but they also followed other means of medical care specially on quack doctors. Simultaneously the people were unable to avail the modern facilities in every aspect. Under this situation they were neither getting adequate modern medical facilities nor they were able to practice their traditional medical systems. There were no adequate solution to overcome these problems. The WHO's declarations of 'Health For All' by 2000 AD is far from any kind of proper implications here and it is impossible to state the fact that how long this poor people will be debarred from the modern health facilities. This present situation may be prevented if some health awareness programmes are conducted among them by the government and the NGOs.

References

Dash Sharma, P. 2004. Nutrition and Health among the Tribes of India, in A.K. Kalla and P.C. Joshi (eds.) *Tribal Health and Medicines*. Concept Publishing Company, New Delhi. pp. 71–97.

Ganguly, Swapan. 1982. Calcutta's Rickshaw-Pullers. *Economic and Political Weekly*, 17 (41): 1636.

Michael, S.M. 1989. *Culture and Urbanization*. Inter India Publication, New Delhi.

National Sample Survey Organization. 2001. *Differences in Level of Consumption among Socio-Economic Groups: 1999–2000,* NSS Report No. 472, , Ministry of Statistics and Programme Implementation, Government of India, New Delhi.

Sinha, Nalin. 2008. *Cycle Rickshaw and Cycling Advocacy in Delhi.* ITDP Strategic Planning Meeting Ixtapan de la Sal, Mexico.

Sachchidananda. 1994. Social-Cultural Dimension of Tribal Health, in Salil Basu (ed) *Tribal Health in India*. Manak Publications Pvt. Ltd., New Delhi. pp. 57–69.

Tauhidul, M. Anwar. 1995. *Rickshaw Pullers in Dhaka City: Their Problems and their Perception about Certain Common Issues*. Poll paper 1, Centre for Analysis and Choice, Dhaka.

United Nations Development Programme. 2003. *Human Development Report*. Oxford University Press, New York.

Warren, Jim. 1994. Living on the Razor's Edge: The Rickshaw Men of Singapore between Two Wars. *Bulletin of Concerned Asian Scholars*, 16 (4): 38–51.

World Health Organization. 1948. *The World Health Report*. Geneva.

CHAPTER 8

Health and Socio-Economic Status of Rag-Picker Children

An Anthropological Study

JOKHAN SHARMA, ABHISHEK CHAUHAN AND ALOK KUMAR

The process of industrialisation in India brought about fundamental change in the mode of production and in the relationship of productive factors (Madan, 2005). The mechanisation made agriculture capital intensive. Those with small and non-viable land holding had to give up their lands and work for the richer farmers in the village or migrate to cities for their survival. The industries could not absorb the whole displaced labour, unemployment and poverty compelled the whole family, including the children to work (Soni, 2009). These child workers are engaged in various types of working situations in unorganised urban sectors like daily wage casual labourers in small factories and workshops, miscellaneous trades, domestic services, workers bound as apprentices to artisans or self employed workers engaged in various street works. They have to work in an unkind, uncomfortable and often physically hazardous environment for long hours of the day without rest. They are ill paid and conditions of work are often exploitative (Malik et al., 2002). India has experienced considerable progress in industrialisation in the last few decades. This has resulted in increased urbanisation, a rise in living standards and consumption, and an increase in per capita waste generation (Ray et al., 2004). The unique feature of many developing nations including India is the presence of a large number of rag-pickers who scavenge the city's garbage bins and street areas to retrieve recyclable materials (ibid.).

Health is the most valuable property of human beings. During the time of the creation of the World Health Organisation (WHO) in 1948, health has been defined as, 'a state of complete physical, mental and social well being and not merely the absence of disease or infirmity'. In this context it can be mentioned that health is achieved through a combination of physical, mental and social well being which together is commonly referred as 'Health Triangle'. Health can be considered as 'a resource of everyday life not the objective of living'. Many developing as well as developed countries have been working hard for maintaining the health of their citizens. India is also one of them where many plans and programmes are being implemented by the state and central government for the proper maintenance of public health. Above all, the Constitution of India also has a provision regarding the right to health. But there are many people in our society, e.g., rag-pickers, who are not getting any benefit or facilities regarding health. Rag-pickers can be considered as unskilled persons who pick up rags from trash cans and public dumps as a means of livelihood.

Human Development Report of UNDP states that working children in India make up more than 10 per cent of labour force, which is much greater than the world average of 6 per cent. According to ILO report, in 1979, as many as one third of rural children and one eighth of urban children aged between 10–14 years are at work in India (Ruikar, 1998). Undoubtedly, most powerful force driving children into labour is exploitation of poverty. Other reasons are found to be low level of adult literacy, population explosion, large family, and miserable condition of primary education leading to high school drop-outs, lack of social security and lack of status of child in the society (Malik et al., 2010).

Society, as a whole, regards these children as antisocial elements, an embarrassment to the community, and unfit to live (Madan, 2005). However their useful contribution to society and ecology is little understood and generally ignored. The waste collected by these children is recycled and produces 25 per cent of writing paper, the packing materials, egg trays, economical plastic and household metal items, etc., used in our homes. This benefits society and word ecology enormously by the production of cheaper household goods, and the slowing down of the destruction of the already threatened rainforests. It also helps to prevent the mountains of putrefying waste materials from building up in city centres (Mani, 1995). The rag-pickers' valuable contribution to society should not be ignored and taken for granted.

Rag-picker Children of India

The growth of Indian cities is attributed to both migration from rural areas and to an increase in urban population due to better health care (ibid.). Arising at dawn, the rag-picker children start their rounds. With feet bare and backs aching, they carry the heavy gunny bags that contain the day's pickings. Sometimes they travel on foot over 5 kilometres each day for the choice picking. Their clothing is filthy, tattered, ill-fitted, and wholly inadequate for weather protection.

Most of the rag-pickers are extremely poor, illiterate, and belong to rural immigrant families (Madan, 2005; Mehta, 1985; Sinha, 1991; Srivastava, 2008). Many commence their profession at the age of five to eight years. Most of them never attend any school or have any formal education, as they earn for their families for extra income as needed. While collecting rag they are subjected to contact chemical poisons and catch infections. Because of malnutrition they suffer from retarded growth and anaemia. The rag-pickers are very susceptible to diseases like tuberculosis and cancer due to their exposure to hazardous materials (Kamat, 1999). In most cases, there are middlemen who engage these children. They are required to collect, bottles, plastic, metal parts, glass pieces, and alike. They also collect food-waste for their consumption.

The people picking through the waste come in several types: there are those who go door to door, collecting and disposing of waste from individual home; there are the rag-picker's children who collect waste left on the road; and there are whole families who make their living by sifting through urban dumps to reclaim garbage. There are two types of scrap-collectors: the rag-pickers, mostly women, small children who collect garbage on dumping grounds, in residential areas or in street bins, and the itinerant buyers who purchase scrap directly from households, offices and shops. Most of the itinerant buyers are male and they typically require a certain amount of capital to purchase scrap. Most of the rag-pickers are not independent but work for middlemen or contractors who purchase segregated rag from them on pre-decided rates.

Most of these rag-pickers are young children. As they have no source of income of their own and are often orphans or street dwellers, rag-picking seems to be their favourite pastime and their main source of income as well. They scrounge around every day as soon as the waste gets deposited early in the morning at the main garbage centres. But it is not as simple as just finding the stuff and selling it to the *kabaadi walla* shops. The garbage picking industry has a hierarchal format with there being several middlemen who make the most of these innocent children, much like the organised retail industry. According to the NGO '*Chintan*', rag-pickers 'are unrecognised and have almost no rights to work, despite the fact that they save almost 14 per cent of the municipal budget annually. In a recent survey, it was estimated that there are about 70,000 rag-pickers in Bangalore city (50% of these being children) and 65,000 street children living in extreme poverty (Chaturvedi, 2011). They live on the streets, railway platforms, and in the unhygienic disease-infested slums of in and around Bangalore city.

The rag-pickers primarily collect easily recyclable materials such as glass, metal and plastic, which can be sold to scrap dealers, who then process the waste and sell it on, either to be recycled or to be used directly in industry (Srivastava, 2008).

In India, the garbage and waste products are also increasing in almost each and every corner of our nation due to rapid population growth. Many cities and towns are getting polluted due to garbage being thrown by us daily. Hazaribagh, in Jharkhand, is famous for its greenery and natural beauty it is blessed with. Above all it is also famous for its pre-historic sites. So, to control the pollution from garbage and waste products coming out from our houses and factories etc., the contribution of rag-pickers in Hazaribagh is remarkable. In this research area of Hazaribagh almost all people belonging to various castes and tribes reside together.

In Hazaribagh people belonging to *Bhuiya* and *Ravidas* community are engaged as rag-pickers. Most of the rag-pickers are young children who do not have any source of income of their own and are often orphans or street dwellers. Rag-picking seems to be the main source of income of these under-privileged children. These rag-pickers scrounge around everyday as soon as the waste gets deposited early in the morning at the garbage centres of Hazaribagh. It is not an easy task for these children to find the stuff and selling it to the *kabadiwala* shops. The garbage picking industry also functions in a similar manner as the retail industry functions. In this way the lots of profit is kept by the middlemen who are engaged in between the *kabadiwala* and rag-pickers.

Objectives

The objectives of this study are following:

- To focus the socio-economic and health problems existing among the rag-pickers of Hazaribagh Municipal Area.

- To find out the problems of children who are engaged as rag-pickers belonging to *Ravidas* and *Bhuiya* community within the district of Hazaribagh.
- To focus on expenditure of the daily income and the habits like hygiene and cleanliness among the children engaged in rag-picking.
- The major objective is to keep the child away from work and make the people aware of this serious problems and issues.
- To give some suggestions to government and NGOs to provide the facilities to the children and their families with a better alternative to keep them away from work on the dumping ground.

Most studies identified that rag-pickers constitute disadvantaged and vulnerable segments of the population (Kamat, 1999; Mehta, 1985; Malik et. al., 2002; Ray et. al., 2004; Simon, 2010; Sinha, 1991; Srivastava, 2008). Third World rag-pickers face multiple hazards and problems. The participation of children in economic activities reflects the socio-economic status of the nation. The poorer the nation, there is likelihood the large number of its children are found in work places rather in schools. Children are required to work to supplement their family income or acquire skills to become self employed or independent persons (Soni, 2009). While child labour is a product of poverty, illiteracy and ignorance of parents, child labour is the result of many complex issues. Due to their daily contact with garbage, rag-pickers are usually associated with dirt, disease, squalor, and perceived as a nuisance, a symbol of backwardness, and even as criminals. They survive in a hostile physical and social environment. This study shows that the life of the rag-pickers is very miserable and they are engaged in this work for their livelihood. This could provide new dimensions in the research works being conducted in the field of rag-picking within the state of Jharkhand.

Study Area and Methods

The district of Hazaribagh forms the north-eastern portion of the Chotanagpur Division and lies between 23° 25' and 24° 48'

North latitude and 84° 29' and 86° 38' East longitude. Its area is 7,016 square miles. The principal town and administrative headquarters is Hazaribagh. The town and the district take their name from the mango grove at *Hazari,* one of the villages which make up the town of Hazaribagh. Hazaribagh, that literally means a *'thousands baghs',* is situated in the centre of Chotanagpur plateau at a height of 2019 feets above sea level.

The present cross-sectional study observations on the rag-picking children who work within various municipal wards of Hazaribagh town. In this study, the data has been collected through the field work from October to December 2009. Randomly 25 rag-picking children have been selected for this study. Out of 25 respondents, 18 are boys and 7 are girls. They work within the municipal area of Hazaribagh ward no. 3 and 21. The main reason for the selection of these wards was that the rag-pickers within these wards belonged to the *Bhuiya* and *Ravidas* community.

These children have been personally interviewed with the help of unstructured questionnaire to collect the data in order to understand their socio-economic status, their working conditions viz. remuneration, working hours, rest etc. In this study it has been observed, how these rag-picking children are forced to work in such an unhygienic environment for their livelihood.

To understand the socio-economic status of these rag-pickers several variables and indicators were made. Among them are number of family members, literacy level of their parents, socio-economic and health status of rag-picking children. These variables as well as indicators helped us to understand the economic, social and psychological status of these rag-picking children to some extent.

Results and Discussion

Bhuiyas are one of the most backward and discriminated castes in Jharkhand. In all socio-economic development parameters,

Bhuiyas constitute one of the lowest rung of the society (Awanish, 2009). Among the scheduled castes the members from *Ravidas* community put themselves above all other communities of this category. This is the area of major concern that they do not allow the female members of *Ravidas* community to get engaged in work like rag-picking. So the females of *Ravidas* community are not allowed to engage themselves in those works for which they need to go out of the house. Hence they are basically involved in household and domestic works.

In *Bhuiya* community more girls are engaged in the works of rag-picking compared to boys. The maximum number of girls are engaged in rag-picking as they are considered more sincere and careful workers compared to boys of this community. Further, girls engaged in rag-picking contribute more to the income in the family as they are not addicted to *hadia, daru, bidi* etc. as is found in the case of boys. Boys from *Bhuiya* community are mostly engaged in fighting, addicted to *hadia, bidi* etc. and further involved into criminal activities also.

Type of Family

The 25 rag-picking children belong to which type of family is also studied here. It was found that out of these 25, about 15 children (60%) belong to nuclear family whereas seven children (28%) belong to joint families. Remaining three children (12%) are orphans (Table 1).

Table 1

Status of Family Types of Rag-picking Children

S. No.	*Family Type*	*Percentage*	*No. of Children*
1	Nuclear	60	15
2	Joint	28	07
3	Orphan (No family)	12	03
	Total	100	25

On the Basis of Members in Family

The number of family members has a greater impact in the life of these children engaged in rag-picking. It reflects the liabilities of the family on the shoulders of these children at such a young age due to which they are forced to work as rag-pickers. On the basis of Table 2 it can be mentioned that about 48 per cent of children belong to families wherein number of family members are below five whereas 36 per cent of children belong to a family wherein members are six to eight. About 16 per cent children belong to families wherein the members are more than nine.

Table 2

Status of Family Size of Rag-picking Children

Number of Members in the Family	*Family Numbers*	*Percentage*
<5	12	48
6–8	09	36
>9	04	16
Total	25	100

Parental Determinants

When we tried to understand the parental determinants of these rag-picking children it was observed that 52 per cent children have their both parents alive, 12 per cent children are orphan, 20 per cent children do not have their father alive and 16 per cent of children do not have their mother alive. In this study it was observed that the number of those children is higher whose father or mother is not alive (Table 3).

Table 3

Status of Parental Determinants of Rag-picking Children

Parental Determinants	*Number of Children*	*Percentage of Children*
Mother and father alive	13	52
Mother and father died	03	12
Death of father	05	20
Death of mother	04	16
Total	25	100

Economic Issues

Under this study it was observed that the parents of the children, who are engaged in rag-picking, are generally engaged in working as mechanic, rickshaw-pulling, labour etc. The mothers are engaged in works such as maid-servants and some engaged in working as labourers on daily wages. Even some of the parents are engaged in working as rag-pickers along with their children. When parents were asked if they were aware of the fact that their children were engaged in rag-picking, 90 per cent of them answered positively. Further 85 per cent parents answered that they didn't get any financial support from their children performing rag-picking work. Only 15 per cent of the parents mentioned that their children provide financial support to them.

Income of Rag-pickers

According to the 2008 study, most rag-pickers don't earn more than the equivalent to one US dollar a day (Simon, 2010). Rising up early morning throughout the year, these children hardly earn Rs 20–35 per day. They are required to collect bottles, plastics, metal-parts, glass pieces, and other items. Sometimes they also collect food waste for their own consumption. If they get food wastes in large quantities they share it with their friends and elders of the family. In this study area, the worst part of rag-picking is that after so much of hard labour and patience they are able to earn only ₹ 10–20 per day if everything goes in their favour.

Education

Most of the rag-pickers mentioned that they never went to school for education. Some of them started attending the school but could not continue their studies due to low family income. Education is considered as luxury for them so they need to engage themselves in such work to provide economic support to their family members. Due to this reason many of the children are working as rag-pickers are not able to join the schools even though schools are situated in their neighbourhood. Some of them never went to schools as their parents are not alive and there was no one to guide them.

Health Issues

Long Working Hours

In this study it was found that about 72 per cent of the rag-pickers are boys and they are eight in numbers. Whereas on the other hand 28 per cent of the rag-pickers are girls and they are seven in number. The age of these rag-pickers are from 9 to 12 years and it is 52 per cent (13 in numbers) engaged in rag-picking.

Generally these children work in one shift but some of them are engaged in collecting the rag two to three times in a day. The shift of these children also depends upon the rag that they collect. As those children who are involved in collection of empty bottles work at night. These children also face lots of difficulties, especially during the winter season. Even after hard work, sometimes these children fail to collect the rag or wastes which would provide them sufficient income for their livelihood.

Hazardous Work Conditions

The rag-pickers are as much a part of our society as we are. Its a rag picker's pride that he is not a beggar or a thief. You will find them almost every where scavenging the garbage cans and the garbage dumping grounds. No, it's not food that they are after, though if they find a half eaten apple or two, it would well be a bonus for them. And it is not just rags that they are after. But they are on a constant look out for plastic, clothes, metal pieces, boxes and a host of other things that you and I throw away nonchalantly every day (Srivastava, 2008).

Rag-picking can be considered as one of the most dangerous and dehumanising activity in India. The young children who are working as rag-pickers are forced to work in an environment in which they are surrounded by crows and dogs under bad weather conditions. They are forced to search useful materials from hazardous wastes without gloves or shoes. These children use the dumping ground as a plain field and they usually work upon the needles, syringes, used condoms, saline bottles, soiled gloves, and other hospital wastes. Sometimes they also get injuries due to walking on the samples of plastic and iron items.

The rag-pickers easily come in contact with the poisonous chemicals and other harmful materials as compared to general people. As a result the rag-picking children suffer from many diseases such as respiratory problems, breathing problems, worms, anaemia, fever and other problems which include cuts, rashes and dog bites. They also suffer from diseases like tuberculosis and cancer due to their exposure to hazardous materials.

Health Related Results

Health is one of the basic human needs and access to health services is right of everyone. Health has a broader meaning referring to a state of complete physical, mental and social well-being and not merely the absence of disease and infirmity. During the study we found that the working place of the children employed in rag-picking is very filthy. Among 25 children on whom the study was conducted only seven children were wearing shoes and slippers while picking rags. Remaining 18 (72%) were bare footed. When asked from these 18 children any fear of working bare foot, 12 (66%) replied that they do fear, but they don't have money to purchase slippers. While six (33%) replied that they do not fear.

Various types of health related problems observed among these children are cough, headache, fever, skin infections, breathing problems, stomach pain, and knee joint pain, cut marks, and itching. These problems are mainly due to precautions not taken by them during rag-picking. Of these problems 80 per cent is related to cuts and skin injuries, 68 per cent with headache and stomach pain, and 56 per cent of cough.

Conclusion

In this study 25 rag-picking children from Hazaribagh of Jharkhand have been taken as samples. The age of these rag-pickers is from six years to 15 years. These children completely differ from those children who are working as rag-pickers at different places of India (Simon, 2010). Most of the rag-pickers are rural immigrants who arrive in India's mega cities with the hope of finding a job. Unable to find employment, and perhaps unable to speak the local language, they eventually turn to picking rag, collecting recyclable materials dumped by India's burgeoning middle class, in order to support a meagre living on the margins of society. While a great deal might be abandoned in this world, little is wasted – everything has a value to someone here.

In Hazaribagh the children from two communities, *Bhuiya* and *Ravidas* are engaged in this rag-picking work. These rag-pickers are living with their families and take the responsibility of their family members. The family type and size of these young rag-pickers have been also given importance in this study. It is observed that 60 per cent children engaged in rag-picking belong to nuclear family and the members in these families are up to five.

They live a hard life as rummage (competing and fighting with stray dogs and cattle) through every filthy garbage heap in the city. All recyclable garbage is collected and sorted. If the day's collection is less, they resort to stealing for survival. If sufficient, they rush to the nearest wayside shop to ease their hunger. These young children start working as rag-pickers from eight to 12 years of their age. The number of those children is maximum, who start performing this work from five to six years of their age. This indicates that due to economic problems and instability, these young children are forced to get engaged in this hazardous rag-picking profession. Alcoholism and other addictions can be considered as one of the major reasons of economic problems among the families of these young rag-pickers. Whatever is earned by the parents of these rag-pickers is spent on *daru, hadia, khaini, bedi, cigarettes* and also in *juwa* (gambling).

These young children engaged in rag-picking are also as much a part of our society as we are, though they are not considered a part of our society. They are the one's who contribute a lot to make our surroundings neat and clean in which we live. They perform their work regularly by keeping their health at risk and without taking any precautions to protect themselves from getting infected through various types of chemicals and materials lying in the garbage area. These young rag-pickers can be easily seen by us every day as soon as the waste gets deposited in the early morning at the main garbage centres. It is not as simple as just finding the stuff and selling it to the '*Kabadi Wala*' shops within Hazaribagh town. As like other organised industries this rag-picking industry has a hierarchical process with the presence of several middlemen who make the maximum profit from these innocent children.

The government has tried to do a lot for the young children living within this town of Hazaribagh. The *Sarva Siksha Abhiyan,* the free 'Mid Day Meal Programme' and many other initiatives have been taken up to provide proper education to these children (Srivastava, 2008). The children who are working as rag-pickers in Hazaribagh town are completely unable to take the benefit of these programmes. These rag-pickers go down the drains, *nallas* and *kudedaan* in search of precious wastes and we as a society overlook this. The government's initiatives to get these children out of this life and to consider them as the part of the same society hasn't really created any impact on these rag-picking children of Hazaribagh.

It's high time to stand up and demand action for these young rag-pickers of Hazaribagh. In the name of modernity and development, let us not ignore the harsh realities which are a part of our society and they do effect us in some way or the other. Implementation of minimum wage structure for them can also be recommended, besides personal protective devices for the rag-pickers like *chappals* (slippers), *dashtane* (gloves) and polythene sheets at the time of monsoon. We are already losing many young children who are engaged in this profession due to terrible diseases every year. At the age when they should be playing in an open area, they are forced to work in the most inhumane and suffocating environment. Rag-pickers suffer from dreadfully high levels of illness, especially respiratory diseases. But health is not, at present, the main concern of the groups that campaign for them. In recent months, rag-pickers in Hazaribagh have been denied access to much of the rubbish upon which they depend.

In 2001, waste picking was included among the hazardous occupations banned under the Child Labour (Prohibition and Regulation) Act 1986. Still rag-picking has been briefly mentioned in legislation regarding child labour. So now it's time to take action for the betterment of these young rag-pickers working in Hazaribagh or else they would continue sacrificing their lives due to this hazardous work. Life's struggles and hardships have made the rag-picker suspicious and wary of kindness and offers of help. He is unruly and disrespectful, always suspicious and on his guard. This discourages the volunteers, who become disillusioned and loses interest in working with them. The rag-picker has never learned the rules and discipline that are demanded by employers, so government employment schemes are not tolerated, and all efforts fail.

Many NGOs are supporting the rag-pickers to gain access to these basic services (health care, health insurance, education and vocational training). They also provide legal support or counselling sessions and help them form unions to speak up for their rights. In some cities, their work has been partly recognised and their situation thus improved (Mehta, 1985). In Pune, for example, thanks to the scrap-collectors union, the municipal corporation now issues identity cards to rag-pickers and offers a limited health insurance plan, recognising their contribution to recycling waste in the city. This acknowledgement can have a positive impact on reducing child labour by increasing the parent's income therefore reducing their dependence on the money their children earn.

A matter of great concern is that due to urbanisation, and the daily increase in cities throw-away packing and waste material, the numbers of such children are growing. The present work exposes the children to health hazards and they also develop social evils and different kind of problems, which affect their overall future development (Soni, 2009). Moreover rag-picking has not even been recognised as an occupation by the census (ibid.).

Acknowledgement: The authors are grateful to all the rag-picker children and their families who helped to get information about them.

References

Awanish, 2009. *Jharkhand: A Disparate Cry for Change.* <http://www.pragoti.in/hi/node/3695>. 6 January 2011.

Chaturvedi, B. 2012. Ragpickers Get Government Nod for Waste Management Practices. *The Indian Express*, 27 April , Ahmedabad.

Kamat, K.L. 1999. *Rag Pickers of India.* <http://www. kamat.com/kalranga/people/rag_pickers/>. 6 February 2011.

Madan, G.R. 2005. *Vikas Ke Abhikaran, Pustak Parivartan Avam Vikas Ka Samajshastra* (in Hindi). Vikas Prakashan, Delhi.

Malik, S., B. Biswas, S.M. Mitra, and R.N. Chaudhury. 2002. Some Socio-Economic Determinants and Working Environmental Conditions of Child Labourers in a Slum Area of Kolkata. *Indian Journal of Community Medicine*, 27 (4): 161–66.

Mani, S.K. 1995. *Addressing Urban Issues through Enviromental Education in India.* Planning Education to Care for the Earth, IUCN, Ahmedabad.

Mehta, M. 1985. Physical Health Problem of Working Children, in Usha Naidu (ed) *Child Labour and Health: Problems and Prospects.* Tata Institute of Social Sciences, Bombay, Series No. 54, pp. 138–49.

Ray, M.R., G. Mukharjee, S. Roychowdhary, and T. Lahiri. 2004. Respiratory and General Health Impairments of Rag-pickers in India: A Study in Delhi. *Int Arch Occup Environ Health*, 77: 595–98.

Ruikar, M. 1998. Child Labour in India: Problem and Solution. *Indian Journal of Occupational and Environmental Medicine*, 2 (1): 45.

Simon, M. 2010. *India's Slumdog Ragpickers*. <1800recycling.com/2010/07/indiasslumdog-ragpickers>. 8th March 2011.

Sinha, S. 1991. *Child Labour in Calcutta: A Sociological Study*. Naya Prokash, Kolkata.

Soni, P. 2009. *Girl Rag Pickers: Struggle for Survival*. < http://www.saching.com>. 10th March 2011.

Srivastava, S. 2008. *Rag Pickers in Modern day India*. <http://www.merinews.com/article/rag-pickers-in-modern-day-india/135059.shtml>. 6 January 2011.

World Health Organization. 1948. *Preamble to the Constitution of the World Health Organization as adopted by the International Health Conference*. New York. 19–22 June 1946. Off. Rec. World Health Organization 2,100.

CHAPTER 9

Stress Manifestation in Women Executives

SWAPNA VIJAYAN, SUNITI CHATTERJEE AND PRATITI GHOSH

The executives are mostly those who are at the upper management level of an organisation and have to perform multi tasks. Their role in the organisation is the most potential source of satisfaction as well as frustration and stress, which ultimately leads to deterioration in physiological and psychological condition.

Since the dawn of human civilisation, women in all social families have taken up the managerial job in the family establishment including food, childcare, overall household development as well as in the hunting-gathering activi y. In the beginning of the 20th century, women came forward in various capacities of managerial posts and ultimately achieved success in her field of work. But at the same time she developed certain predominant but unidentified stressors around her but the subject is still unexplored.

Small scale development, industrialisation, exploded private telecommunication sectors have exposed women executives to complexities arising from occupational health. The newly faced problems are comprised of psychosocial interrelated problems including the stability of work, type and rhythm of work, service condition, job satisfaction, leadership, worker's participation and communication, trade union activities etc.

In case of these women executives, their occupational environment is to be considered along with her domestic environment, e.g., stress at work may disturb her sleep just as stress at home may affect her work.

Objective

The present study aims to determine some of the altered physiological and biochemical parameters in the women executives which would help ascertain their level of stress.

Methodology

A study was conducted among 100 women executives from public sector, with fixed work timings, moderately high socio-economic background and aged 41-50 years in and around Kolkata, based on questionnaire method, which did not include lie-scale. Their nutritional status, prevalence of chronic disorders and diseases, probability of any disease or stress, attitude towards foods and their dietary habits, hobbies, etc. were assessed.

Results

The study shows that the executives constitute a predominant section of the population who are diagnosed with metabolic syndrome, suffering from metabolic disorders like hyperlipidemia (>92%), obesity (>90%) or diabetes mellitus (70%).

They were exposed to spicy-rich foods along with alcohol, explaining the common problems of obesity, cardiovascular disease, peptic ulcer, anaemia, cancer, diabetes mellitus etc. Body mass index (BMI) reveals that 90 per cent of the executives are obese while 6 per cent are overweight and only 4 per cent are of acceptable weight. They are more prone to taking convenient and fast food, which contributes to their unhealthy lifestyle and weight gain. Tendency towards non-vegetarian intake is more such that even the in-house vegetarians become non-vegetarians out of their house.

High cholesterol level and high blood pressure alongwith the symptoms of cardiovascular diseases were found among executives of age group 41–50 years, whereas 15.4 per cent of them showed breathlessness, 15.4 per cent showed hypertension, 3.9 per cent showed chest pain and 3.9 per cent showed palpitation as a symptom (Figure 1).

Figure 1

Cardiopulmonary Abnormalities Observed in the Women Executives

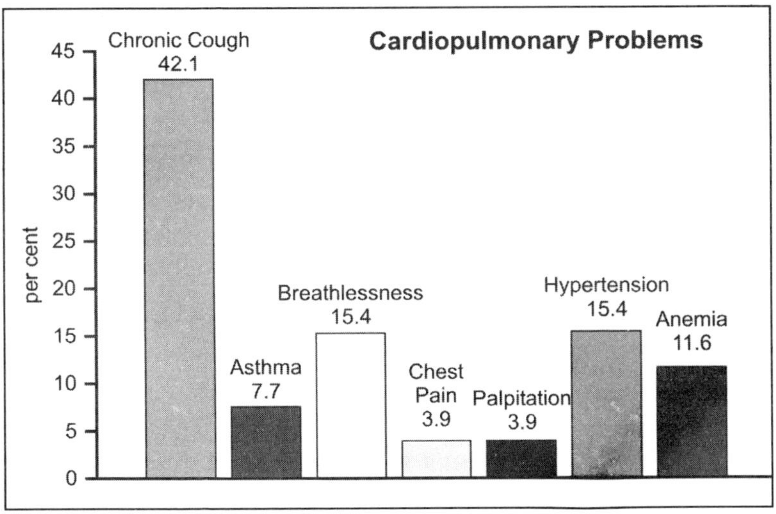

Executives are under excess mental pressure. The symptoms of annoyance (16.88%), sleep disorders (12.98%) and dizziness (7.79%) were more common in executives than the other symptoms like chronic headache (1.29%), tingling, irritation (6.49% each), etc. (Figure 2).

Figure 2

Psychoneural Abnormalities Observed in the Women

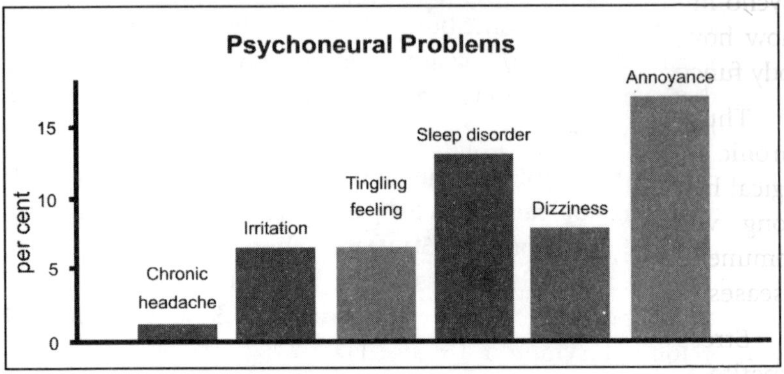

Working for long hours on computers initiates ocular problems. In the present study, 89.6 per cent of executives had spectacles, 8.3 per cent suffered from redness and watering of eyes.

Many were prey to musculo-skeletal distress, especially lower back pain (40.4%) and spondylosis (33.3%) arising from long hours of uninterrupted deskwork, physical inactivity and stress.

Peptic ulcer, chronic constipation and loss of appetite were mainly observed in those bearing faulty food habits. They were also addicted to alcohol, *paan*, tobacco or *gutkha* to maintain their social status.

Discussion

The executives belong to the elite class with high income group usually take recourse to improper dietary habit. It is the job role of a woman executive that supposedly serves as the potential source of satisfaction but it also includes frustration and stress, leading to anxiety, neurotic depression and somatic concomitants of anxiety (Nelson et al., 1989)

The philosophy of relationship between mind and body states that the mental state and physical activities are part of the whole consciousness, whereas feelings and thoughts are epiphenomenon of physical process. Scientific research in psycho-immunology, neuro-endocrinology and neurophysiology show how psychological stress causes pathological changes in body function (Lam et al., 1987).

Thus, persistent stress to attain consistent goals has a chronic underlying effect which adversely affects the physiological homeostasis of executives. This jeopardized metabolism along with altered endocrine pattern, downregulates the immune system inducing a cascade of metabolic disorders and diseases (Adams et al., 2011).

Stress is symptomatised by disruption of sleep, loss of appetite, trembling hands, dizziness and stomach upset. Besides, shortness of breath, tachycardia, lower back pain, ill health and sleepless nights are noticed occasionally among multitasking executives (Alcouffe et al., 1999; Gupta, 1996; Krause and Miyamoto, 1998).

According to National Institute of Alcohol Abuse and Alcoholism, it also causes nervous disorder like neuropathy, dementia and psychological disturbances like depression, anxiety and insomnia. Regular usage of alcohol to counter stress, results in rapid development of its tolerance requiring steadily higher doses. Alcohol affects both the peripheral and central nervous systems (Finn et al., 1990). The damage brought on by chronic and excessive alcohol consumption lead to deficiency of vitamins like folate, vitamin B_{12}, vitamin A and of minerals like calcium and zinc (Lieber, 1988; Marsano and McClain, 1989). Alcohol consumption decreased the levels of cortisol and appetite thus affecting digestion capability (Gill, 2000). Such an individual may be obese but chronically undernourished (Childs et al., 2011).

To avert psychological burden, the smoking frequency of women is catching up with that of the men, and there is a higher rate of smoking initiation among women (Chesney and Nealey, 1996). Relief from mental stress may be sought from extracurricular activities like singing, listening to music, dancing, gossiping, cartooning, etc. (Nelson and Burk, 2000). Exercise, yoga and meditation will serve as holistic therapy encompassing physiological and psychological aspects.

Conclusion

In practice, all these problems go hand in hand with this job pattern but practicing integrity, proper food habits, meditation, physical exercises, refreshing hobby, relaxing in family vacations and if nothing can be workable taking recourse to stress-relieving tablets (Dainty and Moreen, 1996) may curtail the intensity of physiological and psychological problems. So executives should be educated on nutritional value of food, along with the necessity to exercise and relax to create harmonious balance for proper management of time, stress and lifestyle disorders.

References

Adams, C.E., F.L. Greenway and P.J. Brantley. 2011. Lifestyle Factors and Ghrelin: Critical Review and Implications for Weight Loss Maintenance. *Obesity Review*, 12 (5): e211–18.

Alcouffe, J., P. Manillier, M. Brehier, C. Fabin, and F. Faupin. 1999. Analysis by Sex of Low Back Pain among Workers from Small Companies in the Paris Area: Severity and Occupational Consequences. *Occup Environ Med*, 56 (10): 696–701.

Chesney, M.A., and J.B. Nealey. 1996. Smoking and Cardiovascular Disease Risk in Women, in P.M. Kato and T. Mann (eds.) *Handbook of Diversity Issues in Health Psychology*. Plenum Press, New York, pp: 199–218.

Childs, E., S. O'Connor S and H. de Wit. 2011. Bidirectional Interactions between Acute Psychosocial Stress and Acute Intravenous Alcohol in Healthy Men. *Alcoholism: Clinical and Experimental Research*, 35 (10): 1794–803.

Dainty, P.H. and A. Moreen. 1996. *The Capable Executive: Effective Performance in Senior Management*, Macmillan Press, Delhi.

Finn, P.R., N.C. Zeitouni and R.O. Pihl. 1990. Effects of Alcohol on Psycho-physiological Hyperreactivity to Non Aversive and

Aversive Stimuli in Men at High Risk for Alcoholism. *Journal of Abnormal Psychology*, 99: 79–85.

Gill, J. 2000.The Effects of Moderate Alcohol Consumption on Female Hormone Levels and Reproductive Function. *Alcohol and Alcoholism*, 35 (5): 417–23.

Gupta, R. 1996. Lifestyle Risk Factors and Coronary Heart Disease Prevalence in Indian Men. *J Assoc Physicians India*, 44 (10): 689–93.

Krause, D.G. and M. Miyamoto. 1998. *The Book of Five Rings for Executives: Musashi's Classic Book of Competitive Tactics*. Nicholas Brealey Publishing, London.

Lam, T.H., P.W. Lee, S.G. Ong, C.M. Wong, W.K. Chow, and J.W. Kleevens. 1987. Mental Health and Work Stress: A Comparison of Response Patterns in Executives and Clerical Workers in Hong Kong. *J Occup Med*, 29 (11): 892–97.

Lieber, C.S. 1988. The Influence of Alcohol on Nutritional Status. *Nutrition Reviews*, 46 (7): 241–54.

Marsano, L. and C.J. McClain. 1989. Effects of Alcohol on Electrolytes and Minerals. *Alcohol Health & Research World*, 13 (3): 255–60.

Nelson, D.L. and R.J. Burke. 2000. Women Executives: Health, Stress and Success. Academy of Management Executive, 14 (2): 107–21.

Nelson, D.L., M.A. Hitt and J.C. Quick. 1989. Men and Women of the Personnel Profession: Some Similarities and Differences in their Stress. *Stress Medicine*, 5: 145–52.

SECTION III

Changing Health Scenario: Opportunities and Challenges

CHAPTER 10

Urbanisation, Globalisation and Health

A Gender Dimension

PARAMA UKIL

Globalisation is clearly the buzzword of the new millennium but its use is often imprecise (Held and Mc Grew, 2001; Held et al., 1999; Lechner and Boli, 2000). Globalisation is an extremely complex multidimensional phenomenon. It is a double-edged process as far as women are concerned. On the one hand, majority of women in India and other developing countries find themselves stripped off the benefit of social security, government subsidy, protection of labour rights and safety nets. Common people find it difficult to keep pace with the economic crisis and decline in the public sector enterprises. On the other hand, there are possibilities of better education and health facilities, technological advancements and opportunities at the transnational sense which are very attractive to the privileged few (Pearson, 2000).

Review of Literature

Relation between Health and Globalisation

The most appropriate starting point for any exploration of the links between globalisation and health are recent trends in the distribution of income and poverty. In some parts of the world global restructuring has had positive effects through the opening up of trade and the promotion of economic growth. However, in other settings there is evidence of increased inequalities both within and between communities, as well as an increase in the overall numbers in poverty (Navarro, 1998). Under these circumstances the well-established but complex links between low gross domestic product (GDP) and individual ill health will clearly need to be a major focus of investigation across a range of settings. The second area requiring further study is the changing nature of productive processes, which continue to have both direct and indirect effects on the health of individuals and households. Overall, the pattern is one where the increasing power of transnational corporations and the accompanying growth of transport and communications have led to the globalisation of production. Goods are produced wherever it is most profitable and this has major implications for the health and well-being of the labour force and for surrounding communities (Panos, 1998). These changes have meant transformations in when, where and how work is done. For some workers they have meant loss of employment, while for others they have meant entry into the labour force for the first time. In many instances the only jobs available will be located far from home, forcing individuals and sometimes families to move great distances. For most, the opportunity to work offers direct benefits as their wages enable them to buy more of the necessities for health. However, for some, these benefits will come at the cost of exposure to new health risks (Siqueira and Levenstein, 2000). If the impact of global restructuring on the health of workers is to be properly evaluated, this complex mix of costs and benefits needs further exploration in a number of different situations. In many cases these changes in the nature of production have also affected the natural environment beyond individual workplaces. There are some examples of better regulation in the developed countries leading to improvements for workers in other parts of the world. However, in other situations, shifts in methods of production have posed a direct threat to the well-being of individuals and families. Environmental degradation has placed severe constraints on the capacity of some households to acquire the natural resources necessary for their survival, while industrial pollution has exposed whole families to physical and chemical hazards. The third element of globalisation which is directly influencing health is the growth of initiatives to liberalise trade. Working through the World Trade Organisation (WTO) and related organisations, policies have been developed to open up markets and to maximise financial transfers across national boundaries. International agreements have been put in place with the aim of removing barriers to multilateral trade. In some instances this has been beneficial when the opportunity to buy new products promotes the well-being of those who can afford them. But, at the same time, there is evidence that trade liberalisation can cause considerable harm both through the withholding of potentially beneficial products such as therapeutic drugs and also through the promotion of products without due regard for the risks they may pose to consumers (Houriet, 1998).

Gender Dimension of Health and Globalisation

A gender-neutral approach can be used to analyse the impact of global restructuring on the health of both women and men. However, to be of practical value, sex and gender issues also need to be incorporated into the model. Some of the health effects of globalisation will be the same for both groups but, because of the biological and the social differences between males and females, others will be sex-or gender-specific. Models of globalisation are now becoming less one-dimensional as insights from the gender and development literature are gradually incorporated into the relevant debates (Jackson and Pearson, 1998; Marchand and Runyan, 2000; Pearson, 2000). Central themes in this revision have included the gender division of labour, gender relations in the household and the interactions between nationality, race and gender in the shaping of identity

(Marchand and Runyan, 2000). At the same time, international organisations and NGOs have begun to highlight the links between gender and globalisation, with new collections of data measuring the progress of women over recent decades (United Nations, 1999; 2000). These contributions to the gendering of the discourses of globalisation have been extremely valuable. However, much remains to be done. If the health implications of restructuring are to be properly understood, more attention will have to be paid to the relations between women and men across a range of communities. Households will need to have a much higher profile in the analysis as key institutions alongside the market and the state. At the same time the gendered nature of health care itself will need much greater focus. Only with a refocusing of this kind will it be possible to develop the knowledge base for a gender-sensitive approach to public health in the 21st century (Doyal, 2002). In the course of their everyday lives, women and men often face similar challenges to their health. However, there are also significant differences between the two groups. The most important starting point for explaining these differences is to be found in the realm of biology. A woman's capacity for reproduction makes her vulnerable to a wide range of health problems if she is not able to control her own fertility and to go through pregnancy and child-birth safely. This gives women 'special needs' which must be met if they are to realise their potential for health. However, social differences are also important in shaping male and female patterns of health and illness. All cultures assign specific characteristics to women and to men. These include a range of responsibilities and duties as well as varying entitlements to social and economic resources. As a result, men and women in the same communities or households often lead quite different lives, exposing them to different risks and offering them differential access to health and health care (ibid.).

In many (but again not all) societies, cultural norms state that women and girls are entitled to less than their male counterparts (Messer, 1997). This will apply not only to money but to a wide range of other resources including food, land, credit, time, status, health care, and physical security. Although the nature of this gender bias varies markedly between communities, it is clear that in many settings it exerts a powerful influence on who gets what. In poor households women may end up being the most deprived of all, while even in more affluent families gender bias may push women into invisible poverty. These gendered dimensions of deprivation take on a particular significance when they are set against the division of labour that still prevails in most households. Across a range of different cultures, work in the domestic arena continues to be seen as primarily the duty of women. Under these circumstances, the insecurity that often accompanies restructuring becomes an additional burden that bears on women most severely. The most immediate effects of poverty on many women are probably physical and psychological exhaustion as they struggle to weave their own and their families' survival strategies in what are often hostile environments (Avorti and Walters, 1999). This heightens their vulnerability to a range of other health problems, which may often be cumulative in their effects. During the reproductive years in particular, the demands on women may be high while food may be in short supply. This can contribute to iron-deficiency anaemia, which increases women's susceptibility to pregnancy-related disorders as well as to a range of infectious diseases. The gendered links between health, poverty and global restructuring can be illustrated with particular clarity through the HIV/AIDS epidemic (Fair, 2000). This began as a disease primarily affecting gay men in the developed countries but has become a major killer of poor women. In 2000 more that 1.3 million women died from AIDS and there are now more than 16.4 million women living with HIV/AIDS (UNIFEM, 2001). Over the past three years the proportion of women among those who are HIV positive has risen from 41 per cent to 47 per cent. The reasons behind this shift in the epidemiology of the disease are complex, but often poverty is the context within which infection occurs. In a situation where they have few options for supporting themselves, many women may feel compelled to stay with a male partner even when this is putting their life at risk (Horton, 1996). A refusal to participate in unsafe sex may mean the withdrawal of material support, leaving a woman and her children with no alternative means of survival. For some, paid sex work may be the only source of income and adolescent girls are particularly at risk in such circumstances. This reflects their greater biological vulnerability but also their lack of alternative means of subsistence where the rapidity of global restructuring has cut away the support networks that previously existed even in impoverished communities. Alongside the risks of a difficult pregnancy or contracting a sexually transmitted disease, women in poor households are also more vulnerable to intentional injury (Panos, 1998).

Urbanisation and its Effects on Women

Urbanisation has come to represent both the presence of people and processes of production around cities and towns, and the process through which people become urban dwellers, with all its social and psychological consequences. The many theories of urbanisation reinforce the fact that urbanisation is fuelled by a number of different factors such as poverty, the search for employment, loss of tenure of land in rural areas, and changes in farming and service industries. A rural urban inequality is formed as a result of urbanisation. The process of urbanisation is increasing the economic barrier and results in migration. This increases the regional inequality. Industrial development takes place due to free flow of commodities and capital which affects the production process. Gender perspective on hazards in the workplace and in the community like poverty, the urbanisation of production has also been gendered in its causes and effects. Changes in the way goods and services are produced have not been uniform and have varied markedly between regions countries, and communities. However, they have often had a particular impact on the health of women because of their increasing involvement in waged work, as well as through the changes that have occurred in patterns of subsistence and domestic labour (Chhachhi and Pittin, 1996). Women's work is increasingly combined with child-bearing and in many parts of the world it is undertaken in the informal sector. However, it has rarely been balanced by men taking on a significantly larger share of domestic responsibilities (UN, 2000). Hence many women have experienced a major increase in the overall volume of the duties they are expected to carry out. The waged work can offer women important advantages in terms of both material and social support (Doyal, 2002). However, the nature of their working conditions and the way the work is organised mean that for many these advantages have to be paid for by threats to health. Globalisation has seen an increasing demand for flexible labour forces that will meet employers' needs at the lowest possible cost. Frequently these will be made up of women in countries with weak regulatory regimes who are less likely to be unionised and more willing to work for low wages. Under these circumstances female workers may face both new and old hazards, especially in the Export Processing Zones (EPZs) where they usually make up the majority of the workforce. In the electronics industry young women are often exposed to a multiplicity of toxic substances with complex and chronic effects on their health. The increase in the incidence of repetitive strain injury (RSI) among those working at computer terminals and other high speed machines offers another example of new hazards associated with what have traditionally been female jobs. It is important that these new risks associated with 'modern' technologies are given appropriate attention. Nevertheless, the hazards most commonly faced by poor women are still the more traditional ones found in old industries such as textiles or in the informal sector where so many of them eke out a precarious living (Delahanty and Shefali, 1999; UN, 2000). The work they are called upon to perform is often strenuous, monotonous and ergonomically unsound. In addition, many report gender-specific problems such as sexual harassment or even violence. For those who work at home, the pressures of combining waged labour and childcare can be intense and for most the monetary rewards are very low (Chen et al., 1999). Despite the widespread perception of home as a sanctuary it is clear that many women face growing hazards in the course of their domestic labours. These include the huge burden of lung disease suffered by women as result of pollution from cooking stoves (Sims and Butter, 2000). In some areas this is increasing as supplies of fuelwood diminish and other sources of energy have to be used which increase the length of cooking time as well as levels of pollution. In rural areas women may also experience especially high levels of exposure to pesticides, both through their work in the fields and also because of the storage of these and other chemicals inside or near the home. Because of their responsibilities for a range of subsistence activities it is often women who are most affected by environmental degradation.

Opening up of Markets, Benefits and Risks for Women

The opening up of world markets has created a range of new possibilities for both male and female consumers but again the effects can be differentiated by gender. On the plus side, new products have theoretically become available to those who might benefit from them. But on the negative side, those in greatest need may not be able to afford them. The potentially negative effects of liberalisation for women in particular can be seen in the case of two very different commodities: pharmaceuticals and tobacco (Samet and Yoon, 2001). Pharmaceuticals will usually be of benefit to those for whom they are appropriately prescribed. It is when they are unattainable that serious problems arise. This is evident in many of the world's poorest countries where Trade Related Intellectual Property Rights (TRIPS) agreements have protected the profits of the industry but left potential consumers without access to products that could improve their health or even save their lives (Mirza, 1999). These hazards are exacerbated when inferior drugs which cannot be sold at home are exported to those countries with less effective regulation. While both women and men are affected by these trends, there are good reasons for assuming that the impact on women might be especially severe. In the first place, the high cost of potentially beneficial drugs will hit those with the fewest resources and the lowest social status hardest. In many situations this is likely to be women. In the context of low quality or untested drugs, again it is women who are likely to be most at risk. There are many accounts from those working in reproductive health of drugs and devices that cannot be used in the developed countries but are dumped on those with little choice. Poor women have also been used as captive populations to test contraceptives and other drugs that they may never be able to afford for themselves. In the case of tobacco marketing we can see that again both women and men may be at risk. However, the current epidemic of smoking-related diseases is clearly a highly gendered one. Global estimates suggest that around 12 per cent of women now smoke, compared with 48 per cent of men (Samet and Yoon, 2001). This ratio is likely to change dramatically in the near future since smoking is already increasing rapidly among young women in many parts of the world.

Discussion

The current wave of globalisation has a profound impact on the mental health and well-being of people worldwide that has largely gone unmeasured. Rapid economic restructuring, financial crisis and economic insecurity, the increase in conflict worldwide, changes to social safety nets, and distinct patterns of migration and urbanisation have contributed to social and familial fragmentation. This has adverse impact on mental health of people. The women and children are the worst sufferers. This is particularly true among the poorest and most marginalised segments of a given society, namely women and children from ethnic minorities, internally displaced persons, asylum seekers and refugees. Adverse mental health outcomes frequently associated with these conditions include an increase in the incidence of gender-based violence, sexual violence and trafficking, ethnic conflict, addictions (alcohol and illicit drugs) particularly in men and boys; as well as depression, anxiety and post-traumatic stress disorder more commonly found in women and girls.

The current trend of urbanisation exacerbates existing inequities and inequalities and contributes to conditions associated with violence and discrimination. Caste based discrimination and social restrictions, inadequate access to productive resources, insufficient advancement facilities and powerlessness act as contributing factors to these inequalities (Banerjee-Guha, 2002).

All the above factors adversely impact the health, development and productivity of individuals. Notably, poor women and children in developing countries appear to be at greatest risk. The significant impacts of urbanisation and globalisation on women's health are the theme of this paper. Several declarations and targets are there for improving the condition of women's health. But there is question regarding their implementation. The Millennium Development Goals of the United Nations is one of them which focuses on health, education, development, environmental sustainability etc. The targets regarding women's health concentrates only on the maternal health, maternal mortality and communicable diseases of women (Basu, 2005) like HIV/AIDS, malaria, tuberculosis. It does not emphasise on mental health, sexual health of adolescents, different gynecological problems and other primary health rights of women. Female foeticide is a burning issue in some of the developing countries where the rights of unborn are violated. (Raghupathy, 1997). Women's right to health is violated even before they are born. The goals and targets should be formulated in such a manner so that they can cater the needs of all categories of women. There is no mention of mental health, female foeticide, sexual health of adolescents and non-mothers and primary health rights of women which are deeply influenced by urbanisation. To ensure the right to health of women these targets should be included and a gender sensitive approach has to be developed for combating the harmful effects of urbanisation and globalisation.

Case Study Analysis

The above points can be illustrated with examples of four case studies.

The first case study is of a woman of 18 years. She is single and stays at Purpat, Udaynarayanpur in West Bengal. She stays with her parents and two siblings. She was suffering from menorrhagia which is abnormally heavy or prolonged menstruation and irregular menstruation. Her average duration of menstrual problem is eight days. Her last menstrual period occurred in 18 September 2010. She was suffering from severe abdominal pain for the last five days. During the interview she once admitted that she is having a physical relationship with her boyfriend who stays in her neighbourhood. She did not disclose anything more about this affair and said that she wants to marry this particular guy after he gets a good respectable job. Her parents are unaware of this relationship. She was admitted to the hospital after one week of suffering. Cyst was found on her right ovary and scars were also present in her vagina which remains untreated. Exploratory laparotomy (surgical procedure involving a large incision through the abdominal wall) will be done for further investigation. It was also found that she was suffering from hypertension. The incision was done successfully and now the patient is doing well.

The sexual health of adolescents is not addressed in the Millennium Development Goals (MDGs). Here we found a girl who is sexually active and suffers from sexual complications. She has the freedom to go outside and interact with people of her own age group. Her boyfriend migrated from village in search of better job opportunity and stayed in her locality. The process of migration is an outcome of urbanisation which has encouraged many young people to migrate at the cities for better career prospects. The respondent had an affair with this man and had an intimate physical relationship. But she could not disclose to her parents. She had painful intercourse, suffered from irregular menstruation. But she did not visit the doctor in fear of the society and lack of awareness regarding her health. She was diagnosed with cyst in her right ovary and vaginal scars. Thus her primary health rights and sexual health rights have been neglected. If she was aware about her right to health she could have visited the hospital earlier. The topic of sexual health is still a taboo for many people, that is why she could not discuss her problems with her parents. But to overcome the problem of adolescent health the society, parents and the peer group play an important part. Urbanisation affects the sexual health problems of adolescents which are not addressed in the MDG. Only the adolescent pregnancy is mentioned.

The second case study is of an adolescent girl of 16 years old and stays near Sealdah. She lives with her parents. Her elder sister is 21 years old and got married two years back. The respondent had sexual relation with a boy five years elder to her. He is an assistant of a lorry driver and visits frequently to the Sealdah area. The respondent has symptoms of genital itching, burning, pain in abdomen and painful blisters in genital areas. The doctors conducted certain blood tests and she was diagnosed with genital herpes. It can be transmitted through close personal contact such as sexual contact. The infected person usually develops one or more painful blisters in the anal or genital areas that eventually ulcerate and heal over a period of a few weeks. She had genital itching, burning, vaginal discharge and feeling of pressure in the abdomen. She suffered for more than a month and came to the hospital. She was admitted on the same day. There is no cure for genital herpes, although prescription of antiviral medications are available that may shorten or even prevent outbreaks and help prevent transmission of the virus to others. Doctors said that the outbreaks of genital herpes may occur at any time following the initial infection, and these produce similar skin lesions as seen in the initial infection. She was admitted for two days and was prescribed some regular medicines. She was also advised not to indulge herself in unprotected sexual activities.

In this particular case her right to health and the MDG targets are not satisfied. The respondent is not aware of her sexual health. She did not take any precautions and had intercourse with the boy whose whereabouts she hardly knew. She could not discuss her problems with her parents in shame and fear. She disclosed the issue to her elder sister who took her to the hospital. Her sister managed her parents by saying that her younger sister had some stomach ailments. That is why she needed to be admitted to the hospital. Her parents are not well educated. The father is a salesman who supplies biscuits in local shops. The mother did not have any decision making role and control over the household. Her parents came to visit the respondent in the hospital without knowing the fact that she had sexually transmitted disease. The vulnerability and fear of the respondent is revealed here. She was lucky that she got the support of her sister whose husband was also very helpful in this regard. The respondent was also feeling very helpless because the boy with whom she had a relationship was not seen in that area for few months. She had his mobile number which she found switched off. She wants to graduate and get a job before getting married. The doctors gave assurance that she can lead normal life, can get married and have children without complications. Sex education is very important among the adolescents otherwise they can get into troubles. There is an unmet need of modern contraception among adolescent women for avoiding unintended pregnancies and sexually transmitted diseases.

The third case study is of a woman of 17 years. She was admitted to the hospital in August 2011 by her parents. For the past few months her body weight was decreasing. She was feeling highly depressed and suffered from tremendous vaginal bleeding. She complained about her health to her mother when she could not bear the trauma. Her mother was initially very frightened and took her to the doctor. The doctor examined her and immediately suggested to admit her to the hospital. She had medical checkup, there were vaginal scars which was healed during her stay. She was coerced into sex and abused. She was also diagnosed with sexually transmitted diseases and vaginal infections for which proper treatment was needed. Her case history was quite traumatic. Her distant maternal uncle came to her place quite often. In the absence of her parents he sexually harassed her. He also invited her for sex and said if she resisted he will tell her parents about this issue. He will tell that she has provoked him. She was forced into sex which was followed by sexual violence. She was bitten and abused but she did not tell anything out of fear.

This is a clear violation of right to health and her sexual rights are also not ensured. Sexual violence is a pervasive global problem with significant consequences for the physical and psychological health of victims. It has increased as a result of urbanisation and free mixing of young people. Yet in many places around the world, available services do not meet the needs of survivors. There are medical, psychological and forensic needs of survivors of sexual assault. In this particular case the respondent is not married yet she does not have any control over her body. She could not protest out of fear and shame. She suffered silently and felt guilty about herself as if she is the one to be blamed. She was convinced that her parents will blame her for the consequences. Her health was sacrificed due to this. She suffered lot of pain, brutality and sexual violence. Her mental health was also affected. It will take a long time for her full recovery. Unmarried adolescent women are more vulnerable compared to married adolescents. In this patriarchal society they are filled with shame, guilt and embarrassment in the matter of sex. They have gained mobility and interact with people as a result of urbanisation. But these led to severe impacts on their health. These issues are to be addressed in health policies like MDG in order to protect the sexual health of adolescent in the era of urbanisation.

Another case found on sexual health of adolescent where a girl of 16 years becomes pregnant. This unwanted pregnancy happened due to lack of awareness regarding sexual activities. Urbanisation increases free mixing of people, young generation indulge in sexual activities. Many of them do not know the consequences. They lack awareness of sexual health and sexual rights. Many of them have several misconceptions regarding sexual health and they end up in adverse situations. This girl went for an abortion in the hospital with her elder sister. Her pregnancy condition was not suitable for an early abortion but she had to do it as her boyfriend refused to marry her.

Here she suffered both physically and emotionally. Both her physical and mental health was not protected. These issues should be kept in mind while developing health policies. Impacts of urbanisation on women's health should be included in health policies.

Conclusion

There is need for a continuing reformulation of the discourses within which globalisation is described and understood. Existing models will continue to be partial and unscientific unless they are based on recognition of gender as a fundamental organising principle in all areas of social and economic life. There is also a need for more detailed studies of the complex and often contradictory impacts of change on the well-being of both women and men across a variety of different settings. Without such studies, it will not be possible to develop effective policies for promoting healthier societies pioneered by women in response to global restructuring. The new forms of organisations and initiatives have led the way in the pursuit of greater justice. But the problem must be addressed in a holistic approach since urbanisation and globalisation are perceived as overarching process in which simultaneously many different processes take place in many societal domains (Woodward et al., 2001).

Acknowledgement: These case studies have been collected by me from the gynaecological department of National Medical College Kolkata in 2011. The names of the respondents have not been mentioned keeping in mind the research ethics and their privacy. This field work is a part of my PhD dissertation on Women's Right to health and the Millennium Development Goals.

References

Avorti, J. and V. Walters. 1999. You Just Look at Our Work and See if we Have any Freedom on Earth: Ghanaian Women's Accounts of their Work and their Health. *Social Science and Medicine,* 48: 123–1133.

Banerjee-Guha, S. 2002. Critical Geographical Praxis: Globalization and Socio-Spatial Disorder. *Economic and Political Weekly,* 37 (44 and 45): 4503–09.

Basu, M. 2005. The Millennium Development Goals Minus Reproductive Health: An Unfortunate, but Not Disastrous, Omission. *Studies in Family Planning,* 36 (2): 132–34.

Chen, M., J. Sebstad and L. O'Connell. 1999. Counting the Invisible Workforce: the Case of Home based Workers. *World Development,* 27 (3): 603–10.

Chhachhi, A. and R. Pittin (ed). 1996. *Confronting State, Capital and Patriarchy*. Macmillan, Basingstoke.

Delahanty, J. and M. Shefali. 1999. Improving Women's Health and Labour Conditions in the Garments Sector. *Development,* 42 (4): 98–102.

Doyal, L. 2002. Putting Gender into Health and Globalization Debates: New Perspectives and Old Challenges. *Third World Quarterly*. 23 (2): 233–50.

Fair, T. 2000. The Urbanization Process in South Africa. *Dialogue with the Future* 7 (1): 1–6.

Held, D. and A. McGrew. 2001. Globalization, in J. Krieger (ed) *Oxford Companion to the Politics of the World.* Oxford University Press, Oxford.

Held, D., A. McGrew, D. Goldblatt, and J. Perraton. 1999. *Global Transformations: Politics, Economics and Culture.* Polity Press, Cambridge.

Horton, R. 1996. The Infected Metropolis. *Lancet,* 347: 134–35.

Houriet, W. 1998. *The Effects of International Trade Liberalization on the Health of the Poorest Population Groups: Annotated Bibliography*. WHO Task Force on Health Economics, Geneva.

Jackson, C. and R. Pearson (eds.). 1998. *Feminist Visions of Development*. Routledge, London.

Lechner, F. and J. Boli (eds.). 2000. *The Globalization Reader*. Blackwell, Oxford.

Marchand, M. and A. Runyan (eds.). 2000. *Gender and Global Restructuring: Sightings, Sites and Resistance.* Routledge, London.

Messer, E. 1997. Intra-household Allocation of Food and Health Care: Current Findings and Understandings-Introduction. *Social Science and Medicine*, 44 (11): 1675–1784.

Mirza, Z. 1999. WHO/TRIPS, Pharmaceuticals and Health: Impacts and Strategies. *Development*, 42 (4): 92–97.

Navarro, V. 1998. Neoliberalism, Globalization, Unemployment, Inequalities and the Welfare State. *International Journal of Health Services*, 28 (4): 607–82.

Panos. 1998. *Intimate Enemy: Gender Violence and Reproductive Health.* Panos Briefing No. 27.

Pearson, R. 2000. Moving the Goalposts: Gender and Globalisation in the Twenty-First Century. *Gender and Development*, 8 (1): 10–19.

Raghupathy, S. 1997. Unwanted Pregnancies and Preventive Health Care Use in Thailand. *Population Research and Policy Review*, 16 (6): 579–95.

Samet, J. and S.Y. Yoon (eds.). 2001. *Women and the Tobacco Epidemic: Challenges for the 21st Century.* World Health Organization, Geneva.

Sims, J. and M. Butter. 2000. *Gender Equity and Environmental Health.* Working Paper Series 10 (6). Harvard Center for Population and Development, Cambridge.

Siqueira, C. and C. Levenstein. 2000. Dependent convergence: the importation of technological Hazards by semi-peripheral countries. *International Journal of Health Services*, 30 (4): 681–69.

UNIFEM. 2001. *Gender and HIV/AIDS: Facts and Statistics.* <https://www.unifem.undp.org/hiv_aids/hiv_facts.html>. 11 February 2011.

United Nations. 1999. *World Survey on the Role of Women in Development: Globalisation, Gender and Work.* New York.

——. 2000. *The World's Women 2000: Trends and Statistics, Social Statistics and Indicators* Series K no. 16. New York.

Woodward, N., N. Drager, R. Beaglehole, and D. Lipson. 2001. Globalization and Health: A Framework for Analysis and Action. *Bulletin of the World Health Organization*, 79 (9): 875–81.

CHAPTER 11

Changing Dimension of Health Care System

The Toto Scenario

RIMI DUTTA AND PINAK TARAFDAR

Health has been one of the fundamental concerns of man since his emergence on the planet. World Health Organization (WHO) gave an utopian definition of health as 'a state of complete physical, mental and social well being and not mere absence of disease or infirmity' (Park, 2005). On one hand, health is of universal interest, simultaneously disease, on the other hand is the most inevitable biological and cultural universal. Every culture, irrespective of its simplicity and complexity has its own beliefs and practices concerning health and disease. The tribal system of medicines is based on the diversity of cultural practices, traditional knowledge and social organisations. Tribes are relatively isolated and autonomous groups. Their own indigenous knowledge and medical system is one of the important systems of tribal society. Health, disease and treatment particularly in tribal societies cannot be properly understood in isolation. Health, disease and medicine are inextricably linked to the area of social relationships. Social cultural practices of tribes also put some sort of implications towards concept of health. Hence it would be asserted that the concepts of health, disease and treatment are influenced by the concerned culture. The members of a tribal group are generally guided by the traditionally laid down customs and social cultural practices. Each member of tribal society is ideally expected to follow all the rules. The rapid pace of urbanisation is continuously creating an obvious effect on social, economic as well as political life which eventually disbalances the societal structure of the community people (Chaudhuri, 1990; 2003).

The pace of urbanisation is quite fast in most of the developing countries including India. The multi-ethnic societies of our country witness how the wave of urbanisation changes the social structure as well as reforms the institutional values of a multi-layered society (Singh, 2002). Presently about 67.5 million Indian tribal population is facing the worst consequences of rapid urbanisation. The gradual encroachment by the modern society and exposure to the apparently alien modern culture is creating continues stress on configuration of social structure particularly among the tribal population. This eventually leads to the changes in the behavioural aspect of health of a tribal society which is often guided by the traditionally laid down customs and norms.

Location of the Study

India is the second populous country of the world having a population size of 1,027,0415,247 and covering 2.4 per cent of the total world area. The tribal population of India form 8.08 per cent of the total population and constitutes nearly 15 per cent of the total world's population which carries diverse social and religious customs and sub-cultural beliefs. Among the various states West Bengal is well known for its diverse ethnic profile. The total population of the state is 8,02,21,171 of which 4,406,794 belong to the scheduled tribe constituting 5.5 per cent of the total population.

Among the various scheduled tribes, Totos are the smallest Primitive Tribal Groups (PTGs) residing in West Bengal. This small tribe is concentrated in the northern border of the state in Madarihat block under Alipurduar sub-division of Jalpaiguri district. The den of Totos is known as Totopara. Presently they have a population of 1,300 of which 685 are male and 615 are female (Totopara Tribal Welfare Center, since 1990).

The Totopara mouja is divided into six segments, i.e., *Mondal gaon, Subba gaon, Panchayet gaon, Mitran gaon, Puja gaon,* and *Dhumci gaon*. Beside the Totos there were several other communities which resided in the village viz. Nepali, Bihari, Bengali, Mech, Garo, and Muslim. The village is multi-ethnic in nature. Altogether 238 families were covered under this study. The secondary data were collected from various census reports, sample surveys, books, journals, and local health centres.

In the present study all the six sectors were selected under the two broad categories. The selection was made on the basis of distance from Primary Health Centre (PHC), local market, economic status etc. Dhumci gaon, Mitran gaon, Puja gaon, i.e., the Category 1 village sectors are the most distant places in comparison to Category 2 village sectors, i.e., Mondal gaon, Panchayet gaon, Subba gaon (Chaudhari, 2005; Tarafdar, 2010).

The People

There was no proper historical record regarding the exact period when the ancestors of the Totos of Totopara arrived in the forest village. During different field studies none of the Totos could even recollect any folktales or story of their previous migration.

Although the administration has changed several times but the Toto people inhabit in the same area since hundreds of years with their strong traditional beliefs, customs and societal values. As they are living in the area since long, so it seems to be that an effective traditional health care system support them to sustain in that extreme environment. But the ethno-cultural admixture in the village is creating some ideational changes among the Toto people which eventually reflect in the health behaviour of concerned population (Bhattacharya, 1998).

Changing Health Perception and Practices

Tribal populations are predominantly rural (92.2%) and they maintain their distinct cultural identity despite living in their isolation. Although the concept of well-being and the notion of the disease vary between different tribal groups, yet in tribal habitat, a person is usually considered to be afflicted with some diseases if he or she is incapable of doing the routine work which is usually being expected to be carried out by that individual in the society, i.e., incapacitation from work is the universal index of poor health. Thus, mostly the concept of ill health among the tribes becomes a functional one and not clinical (Kshatriya, 2004).

Like most of the tribal communities, Totos have also number of folk practices related to health and hygiene. Certain practices are suggested to avoid illness or diseases while some are prescribed to have better health. But with the emergence of global traits, and as a part of state policy modern medical facilities are gradually introduced in the Toto society. This new medical trend is found to percolate the traditional beliefs regarding health care practices among the Totos. With the encroachment of urbanisation Toto society is also exposed to new medical system. As a result of which sometimes the local understanding is either subsumed or traditional practices get reformed. The pace and intensity of the dynamic interaction between urban medical practices and beliefs systems determines the extent of reformation of the traditional medical system/values. Diffusion of new medical technology among the Totos and adaptation pattern often reshape the traditional medical values of the concerned people. As we know in the tribal set up health matters are diverse and some of these were built-in problems whereas some others were imposed upon them, which sometimes jeopardized their overall development and progress towards a better quality health environment. In this regard the studied tribe is also not the exception (Tribhuwan, 2004).

It has been noted that among the Totos the belief in the interference of a supernatural agency is particularly strong in the cases of their main economy and in the context of health and disease. Different deities and spirits are connected with various types of diseases. Most of their socio-cultural activities revolve around gods and spirits (Sarkar, 1991). They identify the supernatural powers with group of powerful forces and deities which control and influence the happening in the community particularly in the context of health. There are number of village deities who are the general protecting goddess of the villagers. But a number of specific deities are also there who are connected with different diseases. Broadly speaking Totos believe in three types of spirit or deities.

Protecting deities or spirits are believed to safeguard the welfare of the village. Their worships can be categorised depending on the level of participation at the family, clan or community. To illustrate '*Tsa-gDang-pa*' is the deity of the house or the family, the *Chimadora* is the ancestral deity of the lineage, '*Chaisung*' is the ancestral deity of the clan and '*Senja*' is the supreme god of the whole community. All the deities are worshipped as the protective deities of the Toto community (Majumder, 1991).

Benevolent spirits are worshipped at the communal and mostly familial level regularly. They worship or penance of the presiding deities of the various streamlets, which is located within the territory of Totopara. For example it is compulsory to worship the most sacred river of Totopara '*Goa-tee*' for each of the family head for the well-being and good health of the family members, otherwise it may bring disease, death and calamities or misfortunes in the family.

Evil or malevolent spirit and deities control various diseases like malaria, stomach ache, headache etc. For example, '*Pidua*' or '*Pudua*' is worshipped at the community level to get rid off from headache. '*Pidua*' or '*Pudua*' is considered as the most powerful malevolent spirit at Totopara (Sanyal, 1973; Kumari, 2003).

It has been found among the Totos that depending on the symptoms of sickness if the reason is believed to be evil-eye, sorcery or witchcraft, the people always would call their own magicians instead of consulting a western doctor as they strongly feel that the doctors are quite helpless against such evil forces which can only be counteracted by the magical performances (Debnath, 2003).

There was a time when the educated people had strong belief that lots of diseases could be cured only by worship and sacrifices without any medicine. The predominant diseases in Totopara like malaria, jaundice, high blood pressure, gastroenteritis, stomach ailments and tuberculosis were treated only by traditional ways. Sometimes prayer beads were also used to diagnose the origin or cause of illness. Different incantations were practiced for different types of witch-killing. Apart from rice, ginger and *'eu'*, fowl which is called *'fasur'* was another important ingredient for apprising the witch or evil spirit. Various magico-religious performances were practiced for curing major prevailing diseases in Totopara. For example, *'Datintee'* puja was performed for getting rid off from severe stomach pain. For healing skin problem *'lumbai'* puja was performed which assured early recovery from the disease. Any patient suffering from cough and cold was given the root of *'Guirabeth'* tree and was advised to perform some rituals in the name of *'Dipti'*, *'Choati'* according to the type of illness. In earlier days malaria patients were treated only by offering two white pigeons, one black cock in the name of *'Mooti'* which was a small rivulet. Herbal therapy of Toto traditional medicine was also found to be prescribe various medicines of above said diseases (Table 1). The Toto people still nourishes traditional beliefs in their social as well as cultural life (Mohanty, 2005).

But now-a-days the way of treatment is chosen considering the duration of illness and the death risk of the patient. Cost of treatment is also considered. About two-third of the society members reporting sick consulted government health service providers and the rest reported to have consulted traditional healers over the counter treatment and also resorted to home remedies. It has been found that 75 per cent villagers from category 1 beliefs in supernatural interference in health habits, while the scenario in category 2 village sectors in just reverse. There is a strong sectarian differences observed in the treatment of various ailment. As the PHC is quite easily accessible to the people from Mondal gaon, Panchayat gaon and Subba gaon, these three sectors are found to depend on modern medicine in comparison to the other three sectors of Totopara (viz. Dhumci gaon, Puja gaon, Mitran gaon). On the other hand, majority of the traditional healers (both magico-religious practitioner and herbal medicine man) live in the three distant sectors of Totopara and are readily accessible by the people of Dhumci gaon, Puja gaon and Mitran gaon. Accessibility of medicine providers (both modern and traditional medicine) is one of the most important decisive factors for choosing the treatment technique (Table 1).

Table 1

Distribution of Families on the Basis of Supernatural Belief (Regarding Health)

Name of the Sector	*Total Number of Families*	*Belief in Supernatural Power*	
		Yes	*No*
		Ghost/Witchcraft/Soul/Shaman/Spirit /Ancestor worship	
Category: 1			
Dhumci Gaon	33 100.00	32 96.97	01 3.03
Mitran Gaon	29 100.00	15 51.72	14 48.28
Puja Gaon	22 100.00	16 72.73	06 27.27
Total	84 100.00	63 75.00	21 25.00
Category: 2			
Mondal Gaon	24 100.00	05 20.83	19 79.17
Panchayat Gaon	68 100.00	23 33.82	45 66.18
Subba Gaon	62 100.00	16 25.81	46 74.19
Total	154 100.00	44 28.57	110 71.428
Total	238 100.00	107 44.96	131 55.04

It was found from the field study that malaria and jaundice were the most common endemic disease in Totopara. The households belonging to lower income group and middle income group were the most affected by malaria compared to high income group. The poor social groups, particularly the wage labourers who work outside Totopara, appear to be the target group of malaria due to their health habits and place of work. According to the respondents from category 1 village sectors, if a person had a minor illness like cold, cough, fever, bodyache, stomach ache, etc., visiting traditional medical practitioner by him/her is most common. But the respondents from category 2 village sectors opined in a different way. However, irrespective of sectors, for illness such as malaria, tuberculosis, stomach ailment, skin disease, etc. respondents prefer to consult with western medicine man in PHC. A few respondents belonging to upper economic as well as social group expressed their view in favour of choosing private medical practitioner. It can be said that economic condition is an important factor in treatment seeking behaviour. Traditional treatment is less expensive comparison to the modern medical treatment. This was a view expressed by people across the sectors.

Depending on the type of sickness Toto people choose the process of treatment. For example, more than 90 per cent of population responded that if they suffer from malaria they would prefer to take medicines from local PHC. The same population also opined that if they suffer from jaundice they would prefer to consult the traditional healer and will follow all the ritualistic performances. The choice of treatment provider is not only guided by distance, cost of treatment, and familiarity with the medicine providers but also determined by socially influenced customs and values. It should be noted that the people affected by diseases expect relief as early as possible. In the process, some of them kept shuttling from traditional medical system to modern system or vice-versa. This is also corroborated by the fact that a majority of the affected population were found to consult more than one treatment provider simultaneously both from modern and traditional medical system.

Conclusion

It is established that medical beliefs and perceptions have their roots in social institutions and social-cultural values and norms of the concerned community. It had been argued that medical practices are not orderly customs of a community rather they are governed by prevailing beliefs relating to cause of the ailment (Tarafdar, 2007). The universal fact is that all communities face various ailments. They also develop specific mechanism to cope with these ailments. In the process, a set of understanding, beliefs and perception develop for various ailments. However, this is not a static process. The role of state in providing health care services in Totopara on the one hand and universalisation of western medicine on the other had resulted in a plethora of treatment for various ailments among the Totos. Introduction of globalised western medical practices results in interaction with host socio-cultural medical system in Totopara.

It is also likely that acceptance of new medical practices creates a new set of beliefs and perception albeit with a time lag. As the Totos are exposed to western medical values, the system is either submerged or traditional practices become less acceptable for large masses. In either situation, practices are altered but the perceptions and beliefs may still be guided by traditional values. The pace and intensity of the dynamic interaction between western medical practices and traditional belief systems would depend not only on spread of new medical practices and ailments but also on the effectiveness for curing various ailments.

It has been found clearly from the perceptions and beliefs reared by the Toto people that the health behaviour is intermingled with the culture of the Toto society. It had been found that there was a time when the diseases were treated only by traditional way (both magical and herbal). Now this primitive tribe is provided with some medical benefits as part of government policy. But they also practice their traditional knowledge for achieving positive well-being. So they are provided with both traditional and modern medical system. The factor for choosing treatment process in case of any disease ranges from medical events like availability of health services, accessibility, patients satisfaction to non-medical events which are entirely guided by societal norms and culture of the Toto community (Bhadra, 1997). In case of category 1 village sectors (no modern health facilities in close proximity), people were much depended upon traditional healers as majority were living in those sectors. But category 2 village sectors were depended on local PHC because of easy accessibility. Instances of early recovery from various diseases in PHC gained the confidence of the Toto people to choose modern medicine. Despite few specific cases, more or less all the educated people treated by modern medical treatment procedure were satisfied by the approach of the system.

Thus, the scenario is gradually changing. The interaction with the outside world and immigration of non-Toto population of the village Totopara is gradually reforming the cultural values of the Toto people. Urban cultural traits and elements are reshaping their ideology which eventually influences their health behaviour. As a result they imply a set of responses under changing situations mostly in favour of western medical system.

References

Bhadra, R.K. 1997. *Social Dimension of Health of Tea Plantation Workers in India*. N.L. Publishing, Dibrugarh.

Bhattacharya, Manibrata. 1998. *Toto at Cross Roads*. Aparna Book Distributor, Calcutta.

Chaudhuri, Buddhadeb (ed). 1990. *Cultural and Environmental Dimension on Health*. Inter India Publications, New Delhi.

Chaudhuri, Buddhadeb. 2003. *Health, Forest and Development: The Tribal Situation*. Inter India Publication, New Delhi.

Chaudhari, M.K. 2005. The Totos, in S.K. Chaudhari and S. Sen Chaudhari (ed) *Primitive Tribes in Contemporary India*. Mittal Publications, New Delhi.

Debnath, Debashis. 2003. *Ecology and Rituals in Tribal Areas*. Sarup and Sons, New Delhi.

Kshatriya, Gautam Kumar. 2004. Tribal Health in India: Perspectives in Medical Anthropology, in A.K. Kalla and P.C. Joshi (ed) *Tribal Health and Medicines*. Concept Publishing Company, New Delhi.

Kumari, Pratibha. 2003. Asur Festivals, in T.D. Robin (ed) *Fairs and Festivals of Indian Tribes*. Discovery Publishing House, New Delhi.

Majumder, Bimalendu. 1991. *As Sociological Study of Toto Folk Tales*. The Asiatic Society, Calcutta.

Mohanty, P.K. 2005. *Encyclopedic of Primitive Tribes in India, Vol. 1* Kalpaz Publication, New Delhi.

Park, K. 2005. *Park's Text Book of Preventive and Social Medicine* 18th Edition. Banarsidas Bhanot Publishers, Jabalpur.

Sanyal, C.C. 1973. *The Meches and the Totos*. North Bengal University, Siliguri.

Sarkar, Amitava. 1991. *Toto: Society and Change (A Sub-Himalayan Tribe of West Bengal)*. KLM Firma Private Limited, Calcutta.

Singh, Yogendra. 2002. *Modernization of Indian Tradition*. Rawat Publications, Jaipur and New Delhi.

Tarafdar, P. 2007. Health Development: Displacement of Traditional Culture, in B. Chaudhuri and S. Chaudhuri (eds.) *Health, Environment, Development and Other Essays: Anthropological Perspective*. Inter India Publication, New Delhi.

——. 2010. Cultural Dimensions on Tribal Health A Study among the Santal and the Kora of Jhargram Sub-division District-Midnapore (West), West Bengal, India. Lambert Academic Publishing, Germany.

Tribhuwan, Robin D. and Sherry Karen. 2004. *Health, Medicine and Nutrition of Tribes*. Discovery Publishing House, New Delhi.

CHAPTER 12

Health Status of Scheduled Caste Women

A Study of Two Villages of Eastern India

SHRUTI AGRAWAL AND PRATITI GHOSH

The scheduled caste (SC), occupying a low position in social ladder, forms a major section of the depressed classes. They are economically backward, socially depressed and educationally neglected section of the Indian population. This is even more applicable to the women folk. Even in the 21st century, caste discrimination dehumanises and perpetuates as a cruel form. It is rampant in India where 160 million SC and scheduled tribes (ST) exist, of which 49.96 per cent are women, who suffer from immense plight (Census of India, 2001). The caste system declares them as 'impure' and hence they are socially excluded. There is complete negation and violation of women's human rights and they are discriminated as outcastes. Further, there exists economic impoverishment arising from wage disparity in underpaid labour.

Women have not been able to lead a life exactly at par with men despite their urge for equality. Globalisation and industrialisation has failed to bring much change in their life, rather it has increased the poverty and this has unfortunately affected women in every sphere of their lives (Bagchi and Dutta Gupta, 2005; Krishnamurthy, 2008). There is also large scale migration from rural areas to the urban areas in search of better livelihood options. Women are left behind to bear the responsibility of the family in the economically and psychologically distressed state, further adding to the existing burden (NFHS-3). In this context, Swami Vivekananda asserted that the country and nation which did not respect women have never become great nor will ever in future. This obviates that a better newer progeny cannot be expected as an outcome of such suppression.

As per the Census 2001, total population of the scheduled castes in the country (excluding the population of Mao Maram, Paomata and Purul sub-divisions of Senapati district of Manipur) is 166,635,700 which constitute 16.2 per cent of the total population. Uttar Pradesh (35,148,377) has the largest scheduled caste population, followed by West Bengal (18,452,555) and Bihar (13,048,608).

The total population of West Bengal at 2001 Census has been 80,176,197. Of these 18,452,555 persons were scheduled castes, constituting 23 per cent of the total population of the state. (West Bengal Data Highlights: The Scheduled Castes, Census of India, 2001). The growth of SC population during 1991–2001 has been 30.7 per cent which is 2.1 per cent higher than the growth of total population (28.6%). Overall, the State accounts for 1.3 per cent of the total SC population of the country (Bihar Data Highlights: The Scheduled Castes, Census of India, 2001).

Objectives

The study aims to gather general information regarding the food consumption pattern and lifestyle of SC women residing in Muzaffarpur in Bihar as well as Madhabpur in West Bengal, as these states hold the second and third ranking in India with respect to the SC population, only next to Uttar Pradesh.

Methodology

In order to fulfill the objectives of the study, 200 women of 15–60 years of age from Muzaffarpur (town in Bihar) and Madhabpur (suburb of Kolkata), each, were selected for conducting the present investigation. A pilot study was done and after pre-testing, items were modified. An interview schedule was framed to collect the information regarding the general information, food habit, dietary pattern, lifestyle, Body Mass Index (BMI), daily consumption pattern, and such related aspects. The study was conducted between October 2009 and May 2010.

Data were collected by interviewing the housewives. Each respondent was contacted twice or thrice according to their convenience, to gather all the required information as they hesitated to reveal their personal details. Anthropometric measurements such as height and weight were taken to calculate their BMI (WHO Standard) with a weighing scale and anthropometer. Information on food intake pattern was collected by 24-hour recall method and standardised vessels were used to assess the actual amount of food intake. The obtained data were consolidated, tabulated and statistical analysis done using chi square test to observe the difference between the expected and observed frequency.

Result

The study conducted in Madhabpur revealed that 65 per cent of the women of the age group of 35–60 years are illiterate whereas 35 per cent of women of the age 15–34 years are literate. On the other hand, data of Muzaffarpur show 22 per cent of the women as literate. Chi square test (2 x 2 contingency) has proved that their literacy rates differ significantly ($p < 0.01$).

Fifty seven per cent women of Madhabpur do their own household work and do not earn, only 24 per cent work in the field, 13 per cent rear cattle and 6 per cent weave baskets. Some of them work as maid-servant along with their household work. Out of 57 per cent, a few women (6%) of Madhabpur who are landless, disguise their caste identity and earn their livelihood in cities to cope with their pathetic condition as widow or wife of ill-drunkard husband, to save their children dying out of hunger. About 46 per cent of the women of Muzaffarpur perform cleaning tasks, 32 per cent, 19 per cent and 3 per cent weave basket, rear cattle and work as maid-servant respectively. The poverty condition has driven large numbers of women into sex trade to earn for their families (Friedmann, 1996).

Figure 1

Occupation Categories of the Women of Madhabpur and Muzaffarpur

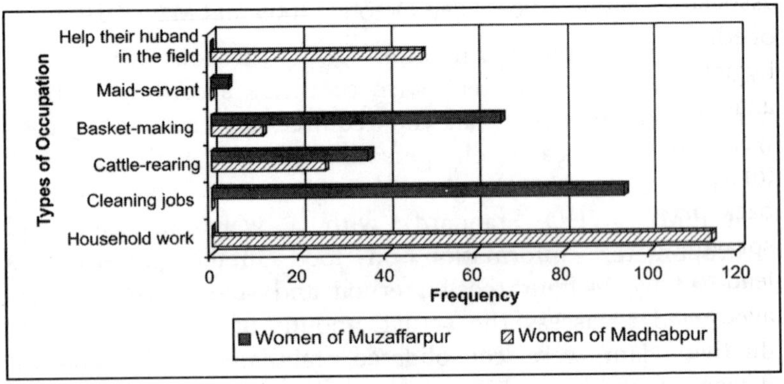

Most of the women of Madhabpur have a small family with two children in contrast with the women of Muzaffarpur who have medium sized family with minimum four children. The girl dropout rate among families is increasing with girl-children been forced to work as child labourers and are involved mostly in hazardous work like *beedi*-making, working in match factories and in the fireworks industry.

The average monthly family income in Madhabpur is about ₹ 4000 but the income is even low in Muzaffarpur ranging from ₹ 1500 to ₹3000 even though women of Muzaffarpur are not allowed to work outside the house due to social bindings. Women of both the places are found to be overburdened with work and do not enjoy even the minimum amenities such as fresh drinking water, toilet, pucca houses, electricity, and separate kitchen. They have a separate pond meant for their use as they cannot share the same pond with others due to their caste.

The nutritional and health conditions are also very poor. Height and weight were taken which was about 152 cm and 46 kg respectively on an average in Madhabpur whereas 155 cm and 45 kg respectively were found to be the average in Muzaffarpur. The BMI clearly indicates malnourishment. Chi square test has revealed no significant difference ($p<0.05$) between the BMI of the two groups indicating that both the groups are homogenous and the contributory factors are similar.

On the other hand, the chronic energy deficiency (CED) is associated with impaired physical capacity (Durnin, 1994). Lack of education and poor status have resulted in poor sanitation and hygiene. Due to poverty, these women are malnourished and anaemic. Early marriage and multiple child births cause the women to suffer from prolapsed uterus. Continuous stooping forward and working while sowing and harvesting cause acute back pain. They also develop skin irritation and allergy while spraying pesticides. Working barefoot on the damp and wet soil lead to development of sores between their toes. Due to lack of awareness and medical care, many of them suffer from reproductive health complications, including sexually transmitted diseases and cervical cancer. The records in the health centres reveal that women are lagging behind men in matters pertaining to medical help. The ratio of availing medical help was1:4 when compared between women and men (Rodin and Ickovics, 1990) which has now improved to 1.3: 1 (NFHS–3). Apart from this, the clinical signs and symptoms of anaemia, phrynoderma, scurvy, scaly skin, lusterless hair are also present in 35–40 per cent women of both the places.

Regarding food consumption pattern, the frequency of meal is four in Madhabpur and two in Muzaffarpur. Cooking is mostly done in the early morning and evening. Cereals are consumed twice in the form of wheat, rice or beaten rice in Muzaffarpur and thrice in Madhabpur in the form of plain rice, *panta bhat*, beaten rice, and puffed rice. Chi square test using Equal Probability hypothesis is rejected showing the difference in the cereal consumption pattern ($p>0.01$).

The SCs of both the states have some similarities in the food pattern as pulses are not consumed daily and its quantity and consistency differ according to the number of members in the family. Roots and tubers are mainly used. Green leafy vegetables, fruits, milk and its products, fish and meat are used weekly or occasionally. Eggs are consumed frequently. Their daily food consumption pattern was compared with the recommended dietary allowances (RDA) at moderate level which is represented in Figure 2.

Figure 2

Comparison of Recommended Dietary Allowances (RDA) with the Actual Intake of Women of Scheduled Caste of Muzaffarpur and Madhabpur

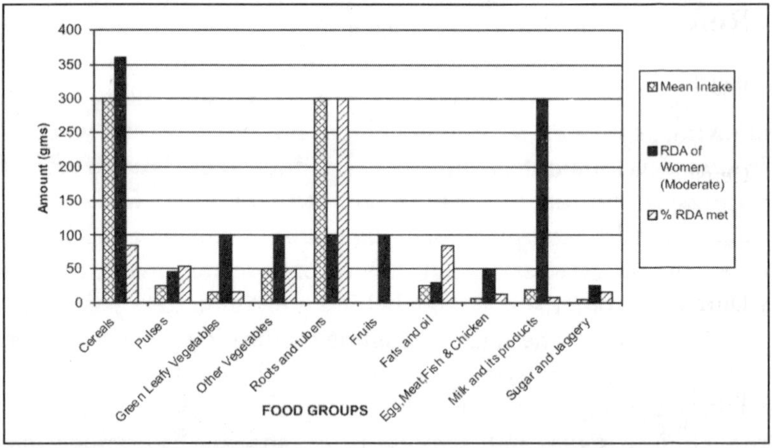

Conclusion

The status assigned to women in any society reflects its cultural richness. The women of both these city-suburbs of the two states are devoid of basic amenities of life, thus implying that the overall social and financial advancement of the states are unsatisfactory. Daily food consumption has been found to be inadequate qualitatively and quantitatively according to Recommended Dietary Allowance given by Indian Council of Medical Research. Being over-burdened with work stress, poverty and poor health, these women lead their life aimlessly without enthusiasm and hope. They toil for the good of the family and children at the cost of neglecting their own health. Various upliftment programmes have failed to bring the desirable changes in their mundane life.

These women expect greater freedom, better education, self-dependence, proper treatment by men folk and a socio-economic environment which is free from random exploitation. A trend of lower literacy among females has worsened the condition. A more coordinated and integrated approach is required to bring about a better living sphere in the days to come which is possible only through education.

References

Bagchi, J. and S. Dutta Gupta. 2005. *The Changing Status of Women in West Bengal, 1970–2000: The Challenge Ahead*. Sage Publications, New Delhi. pp: 244–63.

Census of India. 2001. *Bihar-Data Highlights: The Scheduled Castes*. Office of the Registrar General, India.

——. 2001. *West Bengal-Data Highlights: The Scheduled Castes*. Office of the Registrar General, India.

Durnin, J.V.G.A. 1994. Low Body Mass Index, Physical Work Capacity and Physical Activity Levels. *European Journal of Clinical Nutrition*, 48: S39–44.

Friedmann, J. 1996. Rethinking Poverty, Empowerment and Citizen's Right. *International Social Science Journal*, 48 (2): 161–72.

Krishnamurthy, G.R. 2008. *Indian Health Scenario: Perspectives and Dimensions*. Serials Publications, New Delhi, 47–52.

National Family Health Survey 2005–2006 (NFHS-3). *India Reports. Chapter 14. Women's Empowerment and Demographic and Health Outcomes*. Office of the Registrar General, India.

Rodin, J. and J.R. Ickovics. 1990. Women's Health: Review and Research Agenda as We Approach the 21st Century. *American Psychologist*, 45: 1018–34.

CHAPTER 13

Acculturation and Health Seeking Behaviour

A Study of Kudubis of Karnataka

BASAVANAGOUDA T.T.

Kudubis of Karnataka are immigrants from Goa around 16th century AD; nearly 400 years ago. Stephen Fuchs opines that Kudubis are the food-gathers and hunters in South India (1973: 246). It is little difficult to trace the racial features of Kudubis as it is hard to find sufficient literature and documents and evidences on Kudubis.

Thurston (1909: 99) has acknowledged one of the very factors which forced the Kudubis to move into coastal belt of Karnataka during the 16th century was the oppression and the proselytising movement initiated by the then Portuguese. When the Portuguese captured Goa, a significant majority of them left Goa permanently; those who could not escape from the act of conversion were forcibly converted by the Portuguese. Consequently there are a good number of Kudubis turned Christians today in Goa. Olivinho J.F. Gomes (1987: 79) opines that aborigines stock in Goa is known as the Govddi. The Christian Convert of the 'Gardi' aboriginal was termed 'Kunbi'. It is said that Kudubis fled to the coastal Karnataka and the Malabar regions.

Methodology

The methods used in this study of acculturation and health seeking behaviour among Kudubis of South Kanara in Karnataka are based on my ethnographical work. Further, the anthropological tools such as census, observation, interview and case study methods are used while collecting data. This paper is restricted to the study of health, hygiene, treatment seeking and curing procedures only. Besides, both traditional and modern methods of treatment have been included.

Health and Hygienic Conditions

Ill health has been a major problem among the Kudubis. This is due to several reasons such as unhygienic conditions in which they live; lack of access to clean, potable water, poverty and malnutrition; lack of medical knowledge and information. In most cases, their reluctance to avail medical treatment is mainly due to their superstitious beliefs.

Many Kudubi houses are either insufficiently ventilated or living in joint family without having any facilities of sanitation or hygiene. It is these conditions that have led to various diseases among them. Moreover, Kudubis are more dependent on the magic performed by Gadya. Some of the Kudubis use local herbal medicines or seek the experts of Kudubi medicine man or Gadya. Majority of them do not even admit their pregnant women to hospitals for delivery. A woman during her confinement is kept for 11 days in an outhouse near cattle shed or sometimes in a separate shed attached to the cattle shed. Such habitation tends to result in serious illness or sometimes even death. Kudubis believe that the house and their deity will be polluted if any woman during her maternity is kept in the house. Another unhygienic practice is that the umbilical cord of a newly born baby is cut with an unsterilised sickle or knife.

The Gadya has certain methods of his own practices of magic. He has diverse approaches like finding the will of the deity, causes of the misfortunes and the troubles using both black and white magic. He traces out the nature of the problem, the desire of the deity, identifies the particular spirit that has caused the trouble and settles over the kind of offerings to be made for calling back the power of the evil spirit.

The Gadya starts his duty with a prayer chanting a special verse called *Gadpan* or *Garpan* in a tone that is monotonous while turning the head quickly round for about 15 or 30 minutes. At the beginning and the closing of this act the *Goan* deity, the village deities and all other prominent ones are praised and venerated. The Gadya shows his skills cutting a single grain of rice in twain with a big knife. He counts shells repeatedly. The misfortune due to an evil deity is confirmed if he gets an even number. He uses the plume of peacock at his magical act. It is at this act that the clients take for granted that the evil spirit has taken hold of the Gadya and it speaks through him now.

For years Kudubis seem to have firmly believed that the troubles, misfortune or sicknesses are caused by black magic and it ought to be counteracted with white magic or exorcism through the Gadya. The whole process of the magical act is termed as *Nat* (or *Nimitla*) in Kudubi dialect. There are fair chances that an affected individual might go to an oracle in case the magical act of the Gadya does not succeed.

The age-old superstition bound life of the Kudubis is reflected through their different activities. For instance, spirit worship is very commonly found. They believe that the wound, disease are caused by evil-spirits; they believe that the hunted meat ought not to be sold; chewing betel or smoking, quarrelling over meat are prohibited lest the expedition should flop. Similarly, the liver of the wild pig caught in hunting is dried and preserved in a bamboo reed till the next *holi* festival. It is venerated and eaten up on *holi*. Also, strangely, the Kudubis make it a practice to consult a Gadya when tripped or pierced by a thorn in the bush. Frequent quarrelling in the house is loathed, as they believe that they invite trouble from evil spirits. Omens, good and bad, have a fair share in their lifestyles.

Diseases and Curing Methods of Kudubis

Disease is organic when it affects the structure of the body and functional when there is no visible change in structure, but there is failure of any function in the body. When a contagious disease occur in a certain locality more or less constantly it is said to be endemic, when it affects a very large part of community from time to time only it is said to be epidemic. When an epidemic, spreads over large area of a continent it is called a pandemic and single stray cases of a contagious diseases in a given locality are spoken sporadic.

The most important fact about the primitive medicine is the way in which it is integrated into a whole or a partial, the main strength of the preventive medicine lies in psychotherapy and the sanction that medicine man or a magician carried with him is the faith of entire community.

The diseases among Kudubi community can be studied under several categories such as common hereditary, contagious, epidemic. The common diseases prevalent in the Kudubi community are fever, dysentery, cough and cold.

Hereditary diseases are those which are inherited from the parents. These are considered by the rural folk as the disease sent by the Gods for the sins of the victims not only in this life but also in their past birth. Asthma is the common hereditary disease observed among the Kudubi.

The diseases, which spread from one patient to others through physical contact, are common cold, diarrhoea, skin diseases, eye infection, chickenpox, and cholera. Epidemic diseases are usually believed to be sent by ancestors or Gods as a punishment for the evil deeds of man. It is believed that when Gods or ancestors are neglected or disrespected they become angry and stop their protective roles towards man and thus allow evil beings to come inside the living of the village and give troubles. The villagers under these conditions realise to take vows to the deities and ancestors to get cured. Some epidemic diseases, which frequent mankind are chicken pox, plague and cholera.

The belief on the part of individual is to consider that cold comes from drinking water from different wells or places and due to cold weather and soaking. This prevailing hygienic and health condition about cold can trace back to many generations. By avoiding cold food and cold people certainly avoid further population of bacteria, viruses probably dominated in those cold atmospheres.

In the similar fashion there are many beliefs that prevail among the Kudubi which to a certain extent help to manage health and hygienic conditions. However, there are equally more cases of beliefs which cause further damage.

There are two types of headaches; one is common headache without area restriction and other half headache (*Ardatelenovu*) restricted to specific part. Half headache is believed to result due to disturbances in blood supply to brain due to infection in the nose or ear. It is believed that the fever is caused due to shock, infection, cold, mental strain and so on. When a person gets fever there will be rise in his body temperature. Fever sometimes is also accompanied by running nose. The tongue loses its sensitivity. Treatment involves the use of mixture of little turmeric (*arishina*), cumin (*jirgi*), cardamom (*yalakki*) boiled in water for few minutes and then the decoction is consumed 3 to 4 times for five days. During the treatment, patient should take rice and curry only.

Usually boils develops on the external part of the ear or in the ear canal. The symptoms are ear pain and sometimes puss or blood starts coming from the ear. The most popular treatment for this is thick leaves of Kanbandurali, a parasitic plant, which usually grows on mango tree is heated and juice is extracted and poured in the ear which is giving pain. The other most common treatment for ear pain is using coconut oil heated along with garlic.

The villagers think that stomach problem is due to indigestion and some disorder in the stomach. The symptoms involve repeated loose motions. The local treatment for this disease is a mixture of lime juice and banana given to the patient at early morning or black tea and lime juice. There is another type of diarrhoea which involves loose motion along with mucus discharge and sometimes blood also comes and there will be pain in stomach. The treatment for this is *chakarni beru* grounded in lemon juice paste is given for drink once or twice in the day. If not recovered by home remedy then patient go to hospital.

Kudubi community believes that if they fail to pray or worship *Dyamavva/Durgavaa* and Goddess *Chaudeshwari,* their children will suffer from measles. Child is given massage of castor oil (*oudal enni*) followed by bath of hot water mixed with neem (*bevu*) juice. Every tuesday and friday they worship all goddesses in the village temples by offering groundnut oil to all the deities. During this time solitary confinement is provided to the patient.

Jaundice affects people of all ages and sexes. However it is more common in pregnant women. Jaundice spreads due to dirty water. Mixture of castor (*awdalor*) leaf and jaggery (*bella*) is consumed twice a day for one week. *Naatioushadi* is given on thursday and sunday. During course of the treatment, the patient should avoid oily food and non-vegetarian foods. Patient should take jawar bread and sugarcane juice for one month. If patient fails to recover within one month they turn towards hospital in the town.

The other methods to cure jaundice are toby leaves along with salt are grinded and given for drinking for two days. The other treatment is using mixture of soda and lemon juice. Pepper powder and ghee is mixed thoroughly and applied on the place of wound and cut.

A chronic infection caused by the disease presents a variety of signs and symptoms, depending on what organ of the body is involved. The *Naativaidhya* give *chamurga* oil, used for external application and also for internal administration, and a type of paste prepared out of bile *Karke* (white grass) in lemon juice (*Limberasa*) and applied all over the body once in a day. Normally persons affected by leprosy will not be allowed to stay in the village.

Beliefs and Practices

Most of the acculturated Kudubi societies do not believe in evil spirit but in unacculturated villages most of the people believe in them and are also scared of them. It is believed that usually evil spirits are located in old deserted houses, old tamarind tree, old wells where people do not visit, such places and certain other places like burial grounds and cremation grounds.

It is believed that they appear on dark night of *amavase*. It is usually believed that these spirits attack people. Their victims generally are believed to be in a state of ritual impurity. A menstruating woman or women with just delivered child or a bride who is in pollution or a girl who is in puberty are the favourite targets of spirits. Villagers believe that certain precautions protect them from spirit.

Usually certain diseases which fail to get cured by existing modern methods are considered as troubles due to evil spirit attacks. Most of the psychological diseases which need long term treatment are considered as attack of spirit due to failure in understanding the diseases or due to lack of time to have repeated consultations with doctors.

Once people believe that certain individual is possessed by evil spirit they seek the help of experts with treatment record. Such priests or experts are usually referred to as *Ajja* (old man). These experts are believed to have command on the strong gods and through the help of gods they are capable of restricting the spirits to their original abode. They are called as *shamans*.

Among Kodiyal Kudubis, when a girl comes of age and has her first menstruation, it is her mother and her elder sister who give her a ceremonial oil bath. Some people arrange the ritual of ceremonial oil bath outside the premises of the village temple. Some well-to-do Kudubi families invite relatives and a feast is served to them. This rite is called *Nhane*. The girl is separated for three or five days due to pollution caused by menstruation. On the third or the fifth day, after the bath, she attains ritual purity. However, this rite is not observed in other subdivisions. These rites are a clear indication of sanskritisation.

A pregnancy ritual is also observed similar to that of caste Hindus. It is called *Seemantha* among Kodiyal Kudubis and *Bayake* among Jogi Kudubis. The ritual is observed at the husband's house. The dishes prepared at her parent's house are served at her husband's house. Usually, nine types of dishes are prepared and served to the expectant mother. She wears a new sari and is decorated with five types of flowers. A pregnant woman is not expected to visit the temple from seventh month onwards. This rite is usually observed at both the families.

The first confinement of woman does not take place in her natal house, but in her husband's house. The birth of a child puts the family in a state of ritual pollution. Earlier, the ritual pollution used to end on the sixth day, but today it has been extended to eleventh day under the influence of acculturation. On the seventh day, guests are invited and feast is served which they call *Daval*. On the sixth day a rite called *shati* is observed by womenfolk. A few old women perform a dance called *puguda* holding metal pots. After 40 days, the mother with her infant visits local temple as a part of ritual purification ceremony. If the baby is male, boiled bengal gram with sugar is distributed and if it is a female child, boiled horse gram is distributed with sugar.

Conclusion

Now-a-days, due to the process of acculturation Kudubi community of South Kanara have acquired new modern concepts related to the concept of health and hygiene. If they fall sick, they rarely go to quack or *Naativaidhya*. If they are not cured then they visit nearby primary health centre (PHC), where treatment is free of cost. Normally for small ailments like cough and cold they visit *Naativaidhya*. If they visit *gadya* (witch doctor) they ask them to offer some animal to the evil spirit. It works out to be costly and most of the respondents say that it is unscientific. For major illness they visit hospital. If treatment is of short period they stay there, otherwise they prefer to come back to their village. Admitting a patient to the big hospital involves many procedures and problems. Therefore, villagers prefer to stay back in the village only.

References

Fuchs, Stephen. 1973. *The Aboriginal Races of India.* St Martin's Press, New York.

Gomes, Olivinho J.F. 1987. *Village Goa: A Study of Goan Social Structure and Change*. S. Chand Publishers, New Delhi.

Thurston, Edgar. 1909. *The Castes and Tribes of Southern India.* Government Press, Madras.

CHAPTER 14

Epidemiology of Cardiovascular Disease

A Study in Sagar Town of Central India

D.K. ADAK AND N.K. BAGCHI

Rapid decline of infectious ailments and the rise of coronary heart disease (CHD) as the leading cause of adult mortality can be traced in every Western country since the beginning of this century. Although during the past generation the total rates of cardiovascular mortality have been declining in most European countries, as well as in North America and Australia, CHD still claims every year more lives than all cancers combined. For middle-aged and older men myocardial infarction remains the leading cause of death – or of becoming seriously incapacitated while awaiting the return of the dreaded episode. Epidemiological studies have identified a large group of personal and environmental factors implicated in the etiology of the disease, and diet, especially the intake of saturated fat and cholesterol in meat, eggs, and diary products, has come to be seen as highly important, if not the decisive ingredient in the obviously multifactor disease process (Smil, 1982).

It is well-understood that developing countries like India contribute a much larger share to the global cardiovascular disease burden than that of the developed countries (Reddy and Yasud, 1998). Of all the deaths till now, 25 to 30 per cent are attributable to cardiovascular disease (CVD). This is not a small number. Of this figure, 50 per cent are below 70 years of age and 35 per cent of deaths are in the age group of 35–64 years. This puts the problem in perspective. It is a sizeable problem growing in magnitude. While we ought to focus on malaria, HIV, TB, this cannot be neglected either. As the epidemic expands, people demanding health care will expand. Policy attention rather than resource diversion is the requirement. These figures provided by WHO are borne out by historical precedents. As people urbanise, industrialise and age, this is the pattern of health transmission. But it is not inevitable (*The Times of India,* 2004).

It is revealed from many studies that prevalence of cardiovascular disease in urban India is higher than in rural areas. Krishna and Mathur (1960) in an epidemiological study of Agra, Uttar Pradesh reported that incidence of coronary disease was high in the urban population, in the upper socio-economic classes, and in persons with highest amounts of total dietary fat and highest percentage of calories from dietary fat. Side by side, physical activity was less and emotional stress and strain greater in the patients with coronary disease. In another study on knowledge of cardiac patients regarding risk factors leading to coronary artery disease in Northern India, Uppal et al. (2004) found that maximum number of subjects who had knowledge regarding risk factors, i.e., hypertension was 90 per cent, cigarette smoking 86 per cent, diabetic mellitus 83 per cent, obesity 83.5 per cent, physical inactivity 80.25 per cent, occupation 73.33 per cent, diet 71.2 per cent and alcohol 71 per cent. Average knowledge was found about income 63 per cent, type A behaviour 64.2 per cent, age 56.5 per cent and family history 45.5 per cent. However, the fact is that the cardiovascular risk factors are increasing due to the modernisation, urbanisation and industrialisation. Among the major cardiovascular risk factors such as unhealthy diet, smoking etc. physical inactivity contributes significantly to ageing of the heart as it leads to obesity, diabetes and hypertension. Though there are considerable number of epidemiological studies on cardiovascular disease in different parts of India (Kumar et al., 2006; Kamali et al., 2007; Krishna and Mathur, 1960; Uppal et al., 2004) such type of study is scanty in Central India. Moreover, there is no such study found in any urban centre of Central India. Present study is an endeavour to deal with epidemiology of cardiac disorder in an urban centre of Central India, namely Sagar town of Madhya Pradesh.

Material and Methods

The present study is an outcome of the project, 'Epidemiology and anthropological implications of cardiac disorders in Sagar town of Madhya Pradesh'. In this study a total of 322 adult individuals, aged 30–70 years, residing in different wards of Sagar town, Madhya Pradesh was investigated. These 322 individuals were divided into two categories: (i) experimental group – consisting of 103 individuals who were affected by heart disease. These 103 heart patients were identified from the 2006 record of District Hospital, Sagar, and (ii) control group – the rest 219 individuals, were without any heart problem. For each case age and sex matched controls were selected. The controls were selected after taking the case of heart patients on the basis of following criteria:

(a) age ± 2 years of the case of heart patients in the same age group;
(b) sex matched; and
(c) admitted for treatment other than heart problem.

Data on dietary pattern, social, behavioural and demographic characteristics were collected through questionnaires, while the data on hypertension were collected with the help of blood pressure measuring apparatus. For the sake of analysis the male and female data were clubbed together. Besides this, the secondary data on cardiovascular disease, available in District Hospital, Sagar were collected for the years 1997–2006. This sample consisted of

2,456 cardiac cases. In case of secondary data also the male and female data were clubbed for analysis purpose.

Results

Distribution of hospital admission of cardiac patients is shown in Table 1 and Figure 1 from 1997–2006. It reveals that hospital admission rate increased in Sagar town with advancement of years during 1997 to 2006. Annual totals of cardiac cases ranged from 81 in 1997 to 327 in 2006, with a trend of rising incidence. Month-wise distribution of hospital admission of cardiac patients is shown for the years 1997–2006 in Table 2 and Figure 2. It reveals a trend of high frequency of hospital admission for cardiac patients in winter months viz., November, December, January, and February. During summer months (March, April, May, and June) considerably low per cent of cardiac patients were admitted in Sagar District Hospital. It can be seen from the table that lowest per cent of cardiac patients were admitted in the month of May in this decade.

Table 1

Hospital Admission of the Total and Cardiac Patients During 1997–2006

Year	*Total number of patients admitted*	*Total number of cardiac patients admitted*	*Percentage of cardiac patients to total patients*	*Hospital admission rate**
1997	10,599	81	0.76	7.64
1998	11,099	110	0.99	9.91
1999	11,783	175	1.48	14.85
2000	11,469	228	1.99	19.88
2001	12,401	214	1.73	17.26
2002	12,187	248	2.03	20.35
2003	13,576	327	2.41	24.09
2004	13,763	336	2.44	24.41
2005	15,546	410	2.64	26.37
2006	16,665	327	1.96	19.62

Note: * Hospital admission rate is based on number of cardiac patients in terms of total patients admitted in hospital.

Table 2

Month-wise Distribution of Hospital Admission of Cardiac Patients (1997–2006)

Months	*Years*									
	1997 (n=81)	*1998 (n=110)*	*1999 (n=175)*	*2000 (n=228)*	*2001 (n=214)*	*2002 (n=248)*	*2003 (n=327)*	*2004 (n=336)*	*2005 (n=410)*	*2006 (n=327)*
January	11.11(9)	10.0(11)	7.43(13)	10.96(25)	12.62(27)	8.06(20)	10.70(35)	9.52(32)	8.29(34)	11.93(39)
February	9.88(8)	11.82(13)	6.29(11)	10.09(23)	7.01(15)	8.06(20)	7.64(25)	10.12(34)	12.19(50)	9.79(32)
March	6.17(5)	8.18(9)	4.00(7)	10.96(25)	9.81(21)	6.05(15)	7.03(23)	8.04(27)	8.29(34)	11.62(38)
April	8.64(7)	8.18(9)	7.43(13)	6.58(15)	6.54(14)	4.03(10)	6.12(20)	8.63(29)	8.05(33)	8.26(27)
May	6.17(5)	7.27(8)	9.14(16)	7.46(17)	6.54(14)	9.27(23)	6.42(21)	4.46(15)	4.88(20)	4.28(14)
June	9.88(8)	7.27(8)	9.14(16)	8.77(20)	5.61(12)	6.85(17)	9.17(30)	7.74(26)	9.27(38)	9.79(32)
July	4.93(4)	6.36(7)	9.14(16)	8.33(19)	8.88(19)	10.48(26)	8.56(28)	8.04(27)	7.07(29)	9.48(31)
August	9.88(8)	9.09(10)	9.14(16)	7.89(18)	7.01(15)	10.48(26)	8.26(27)	7.74(26)	9.27(38)	5.81(19)
September	7.41(6)	7.27(8)	9.14(16)	7.02(16)	7.01(15)	6.45(16)	9.17(30)	8.33(28)	7.32(30)	7.95(26)
October	7.41(6)	6.36(7)	8.57(15)	3.95(9)	8.88(19)	9.68(24)	7.34(24)	7.44(25)	8.29(34)	6.42(21)
November	9.88(8)	9.09(10)	10.86(19)	8.33(19)	9.81(21)	10.48(26)	9.79(32)	10.71(36)	8.05(33)	6.11(20)
December	8.64(7)	9.09(10)	9.71(17)	9.65(22)	10.28(22)	10.08(25)	9.79(32)	9.23(31)	9.02(37)	8.56(28)

Note: Figures in parenthesis indicate absolute values.

Figure 1

Admission of Cardiac Patients in Hospital

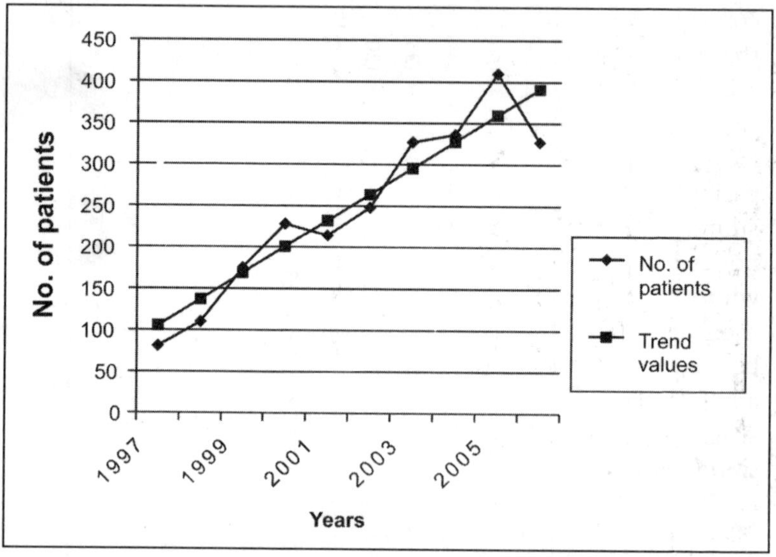

Figure 2

Month-wise Distribution of Hospital Admission

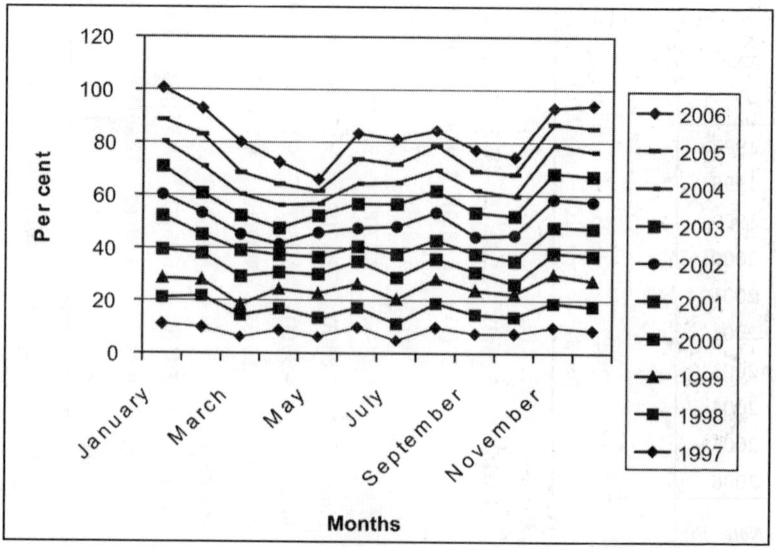

For a clear view of the situation this distribution is presented according to different seasons in Table 3. In this connection data of different months were clubbed broadly in three seasons such as summer (March, April, May, and June), rainy (July, August, September, and October) and winter (November, December, January, and February) seasons. However, this classification is arbitrary. Admission of cardiac patients is found to be highest in winter season than that of summer season (Table 3 and Figure 3). Exception of this trend is noticed in the years 1999 and 2002. Though both summer and winter seasons show lower frequency of hospital admission than their counterpart, no definite trend is perceptible as such between these two seasons. While in 1997, 1998, 2000 and 2006 admission of cardiac patients was higher in summer than rainy season in 1999, 2001, 2002, 2003, 2004, and 2005 a reverse trend is noticed.

Table 3

Season-wise Distribution of Hospital Admission of Cardiac Patients (1997–2006)

Years	*Seasons*			*Total*
	Summer (*March–June*)	*Rainy* (*July–October*)	*Winter* (*November–February*)	
1997	30.86(25)	29.63(24)	39.51(32)	81
1998	30.91(34)	29.09(32)	40.00(44)	110
1999	29.71(52)	36.00(63)	34.29(60)	175
2000	33.77(77)	27.19(62)	39.03(89)	228
2001	28.50(61)	31.77(68)	39.72(85)	214
2002	26.21(65)	37.10(92)	36.69(91)	248
2003	28.75(94)	33.33(109)	37.92(124)	327
2004	28.87(97)	31.55(106)	39.58(133)	336
2005	30.49(125)	31.95(131)	37.56(154)	410
2006	33.94(111)	29.66(97)	36.39(119)	327

Note: Figures in parenthesis indicate absolute values.

Figure 3

Season-wise Distribution of Hospital Admission

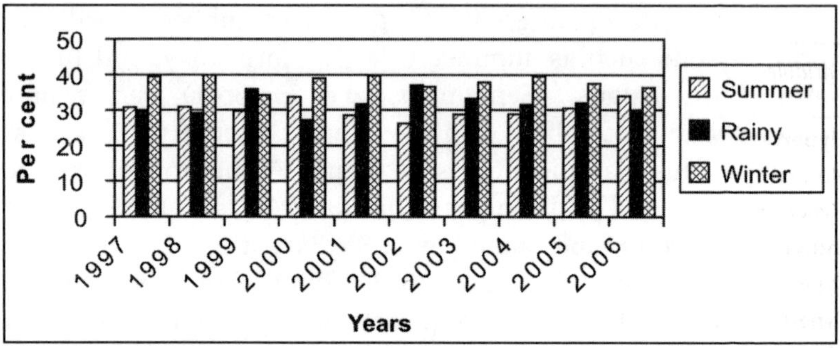

In Table 4 cardiovascular disease is dealt in relation to some biosocial variables in experimental and control group. It is revealed from the table that more than 47 per cent of the individuals in experimental group are hypertensive, while 25 per cent of the individuals fall in this category in control group. In case of individual behaviour frequency of type-A behaviour is found to be higher in control group (44.29) than that of experimental group (37.86). Side by side, more individuals are engaged in sedentary type physical activity in experimental group (66.02) than control group (59.36). In the present study more than 13 per cent of the individuals are having family history of cardiac disorder, while in control group 12 per cent of the individuals are having family history of this disorder. Frequency of illiterate individuals is considerably higher in experimental group (27.18) than control group (16.44). In case of economic condition frequency of individuals with poor economic condition (i.e., low economic condition) is found to be comparatively lower in control group (32.42) than that of the experimental group (42.72). When obesity is taken into consideration it is found that 20 per cent of the individuals fall in the category of obese in both the group. But the per cent of overweight individual is considerably higher in experimental group (62.14) than that of the control group (37.44).

Table 4

Cardiac Disorders in Relation to Biosocial Variables in Experimental and Control Group

Variables	*Experimental group (n=103)*	*Control group (n=219)*
Hypertension		
Normal	54 (52.43)	163 (74.43)
Hypertensive	49 (47.57)	56 (25.57)
Individual behaviour		
Type-A	39 (37.86)	97 (44.29)
Type-B	64 (62.14)	122 (55.71)
Physical activity		
Sedentary	68 (66.02)	130 (59.36)
Moderate	35 (33.98)	89 (40.64)
Knowledge of cardiac disorder		
Yes	25 (24.27)	74 (33.79)
No	78 (75.73)	145 (66.21)
Family history of cardiac disorder		
Yes	14 (13.59)	27 (12.33)
No	89 (86.41)	192 (87.67)
Level of education		
Illiterate	28 (27.18)	36 (16.44)
Primary	18 (17.47)	63 (28.77)
High school	39 (37.86)	91 (41.55)
College level and high	18 (17.48)	29 (13.24)
Economic condition		
Low	44 (42.72)	71 (32.42)
Medium	33 (32.04)	97 (44.29)
High	26 (25.24)	51 (23.29)
Obesity		
Normal	19 (18.45)	92 (42.01)
Overweight	64 (62.14)	82 (37.44)
Obese	20 (19.41)	45 (20.55)

Note: Figures in parenthesis indicate percentage values.

The results of odds ratio and confidence interval of the risk of cardiovascular diseases by the independent variables are presented in Table 5. Variables like hypertension, family history of cardiac disease, level of education and obesity showed significant relationship with this disease. It is revealed from the Table 5 that persons with hypertension were 0.3786 times more likely to have cardiac disorder (odds ratio 0.3786; CI= 0.2317–0.6187). Studied subjects were 2.2792 times more likely to have this disease who had family history of cardiac disease (odds ratio 2.2792; CI=1.2458–4.1698). Besides this, the individuals who were illiterate were 1.8978 times more likely to have this disease (odds ratio 1.8978; CI=1.0816–0.3302). However, the overweight as well as obese persons were 0.3122 times more likely to have cardiac disorder (odds ratio 0.3122; CI=0.1773–0.5496).

Table 5

Results of Odds Ratios and Confidence Interval in Relation to Biosocial Variables

Variables	*Reference Category*	*Odds ratio*	*95% CI*	*Inference*
Hypertension: Hypertensive	Normal	0.3786	0.2317–0.6187	Significant*
Individual behaviour: Type-A behaviour	Type-B behaviour	0.7664	0.4748–1.2371	Not significant
Physical activity: Sedentary	Moderate	1.3301	0.8157–2.1686	Not significant
Knowledge of cardiac disorder: No	Yes	0.628	0.3696–1.0671	Not significant
Family history of cardiac disorder: Yes	No	2.2792	1.2458–4.1698	Significant*
Level of education: Illiterate	Literate	1.8978	1.0816–3.3302	Significant*
Economic condition: Poor (Low)	Well-off	1.4485	0.8947–2.345	Not significant
Obesity: Overweight and obese	Normal	0.3122	0.1773–0.5496	Significant*

*Significant at 0.05 level of probability

Discussion

Cardiovascular diseases are the primary cause of mortality in developed countries and generate a major burden of morbidity throughout the life (Labarthe, 1998), whereas, the developing countries contribute larger share to this global burden than that of the developed countries. Prevalence of heart disease was 8.37 per cent among the urban Kashmiris and 7.4 per cent among the urban India of Northern region. The present study shows percentage figure of admission of heart patients ranges from 0.06 in 1997 to 1.68 in 2006. Alongwith this, values of annual rate of the same, ranges from 0.55 in 1997 to 2.24 in 2006. Thus a trend of rising incidence of cardiovascular disease is very much perceptible in this Central Indian town, namely Sagar. According to Krishna and Mathur (1960), incidence of coronary disease was high in urban population of Agra with highest amounts of total dietary fat and highest percentage of calories for dietary fat. They also found that physical activity was less among the patients and emotional stress and strain was greater in the patients. The study also reveals that admission of cardiac patients was highest in winter season in Sagar town than that of summer and rainy seasons. It is well known that winter is the prime time for heart attacks.

It appears from the Table 4 that there is lower number of hypertensive individuals in control group than experimental group. Besides, there is higher percentage of individuals with type-B behaviour in control group than experimental group. Considerably higher percentage of individuals in control group are in the category of non-sedentary type of physical activity than the individuals of experimental group. Higher percentage of individuals in control group have the knowledge of cardiac disease than the individuals of experimental group. It also appears that frequency of overweight individuals is considerably lower in control group than the individuals of experimental group. The results of odds ratio and confidence interval of the risk of cardiovascular disease by the independent variables show that variables like hypertension, family history of cardiac disorder, level of education and obesity showed significant relationship with cardiac diseases. Thus from the present study it may be suggested that the individuals of control group are certainly in better position than the individuals of experimental group in terms of different risk factors of cardiovascular disease.

Acknowledgement: The present article is based on the project entitled, 'Epidemiology and Anthropological Implications of Cardiac Disorders in Sagar town of Madhya Pradesh', which was approved by the Anthropological Survey of India, Kolkata. Both the authors are grateful to the said organisation. The authors are also grateful to the authority of District Hospital, Sagar for allowing D.K. Adak to collect necessary information from hospital records. Finally the authors express their gratitude to all the participants under study residing in Sagar town of Madhya Pradesh.

References

Kamali, M.A., I.H. Dar, G. Ali, H.S. Wazir, and S. Hussain. 2007. Prevalence of Coronary Heart Disease in Kashmiris. *Indian Heart J.*, 59: 44–49.

Krishna, S. and M.D. Mathur. 1960. Environmental Factors in Coronary Heart Disease: An Epidemiologic Study at Agra (India). *Circulation*, 21: 684–89.

Kumar, R., M.C. Singh, S.K. Ahlawat, J.S. Thakur, A. Srivastava, M.K. Sharma, P. Malhotra, H.K. Bali, and S. Kumari. 2006. Urbanization and Coronary Heart Disease: A Study of Urban-rural Differences in Northern India. *Indian Heart J.*, 58: 126–30.

Labarthe, D.R. 1998. *Epidemiology and Prevention of Cardio Vascular Disease: A Global Challenge*. Aspen Publishers, Gaitherburg.

Reddy, K.S. and S. Yasud. 1998. Emerging Epidemic of Cardiovascular Diseases in Developing Countries. *Circulation*, 97: 596–601.

Smil, V. 1982. Coronary Heart Disease, Diet and Western Mortality. *Populations and Development Review*, 15 (3): 399–424.

The Times of India. 2004. Heart of the Matter. 8 July , p: 16.

Uppal, H.K., M. Joseph and P. Mehta. 2004. Study on Knowledge of Cardiac Patients Regarding Risk Factors Leading to Coronary Artery Disease. *Proc. 91st Ind. Sc. Cong. Part III*, Indian Science Congress Association, Kolkata.

CHAPTER 15

Urbanisation and Its Impact on Health Seeking Behaviour

A Study of Banjaras of Karnataka

V. JAGADEESH

The Banjara who are basically from Rajasthan and belongs to the clans of Hindu Agnivanshi Rajputs Warrior or Contract Killers (also known as Banjari, Pindari, Bangala, Banjori, Banjuri, Brinjari, Lamani, Lamadi, Lambani, Labhani, Lambara, Lavani, Lemadi, Lumadale, Labhani Muka, Goola, Gurmarti, Gormati, Kora, Sugali, Sukali, Tanda, Vanjari, Wanji) are a community in India spread in Andhra Pradesh, Karnataka, Maharashtra, Madhya Pradesh, Rajasthan, Uttar Pradesh and other states of India. About half of their number speaks Lambadi, one of the Rajasthani dialects of India, while others are native speakers of Hindi, Telugu and other languages dominant in their respective areas of settlement. Rathore, Parmar, Pawar, Chauhan, casts belongs to Vanjara community in Rajasthan and Gujarat, now are in general seats after the communal rights took place in Rajasthan for Reservation in 2008, as they were landlords in Amarkot, Fathaykot and Sialkot before Partition of India and Pakistan. While there are other backward classes in Andhra Pradesh (where they are listed as Sugali) and Odisha, a Scheduled Caste (SC) in Karnataka, Haryana, Punjab, and Himachal Pradesh.

Banjaras have migrated from Rajasthan. They have unique settlements in Karnataka. They live scattered all over the state, but they are distinctly identified by their dress and their language. Banjaras are called by several names like Lamani, Lambada, Banjara, Sukali etc. Perhaps the name Banjara or Lamani speaks of their community occupation (Jagadeesh, 2005).

The present study also intends to discuss the four major sub clans residing and occupying its own locality and following its own traditional occupation such as agriculture, carpentry, and so on. In terms of educational, developmental and welfare services, the settlements can be of poor progressive. Since, the settlements in the state were unplanned with very minimal facilities of drinking water wells and borewells, primary school upto class 5 (only in few settlements) and banking, consumer cooperative society, postal and telegraph, electricity, irrigation, and medical dispensary are not found in the settlements. The soil of the settlement is not good for agriculture. About 90 per cent of the population involved in the labour work in the iron ore industries have very bad health condition especially in Bellary, Karnataka. Most of them are illiterates. About 65 per cent of the households live in their own houses and rest of them reside in rented and work as landless labours. Some iron ore industries which are located in nearby settlements are boosting its economy to further heights.

Overall, as title indicates, the present study is about impact of urbanisation on health seeking behaviour among Banjaras of Karnataka.

Methodology

Primary and secondary methods of data collection has been adapted for collecting data. Primary data collection involves method such as personnel interviews, questionnaire and also through participant observation. Secondary method of data collection involves references of books, journals reports, encyclopedia, dictionaries etc. Participant observational method helped collect a plethora of literature pertaining to my research theme and also through first hand knowledge the problem has been discussed and analysed the perception of health and hygiene among Banjaras of Appenahalli Settlement in Bellary district. Being a local man and the fact of my education in the district helped me considerably in having personal contacts and visiting the field for collecting and checking the data.

Health Practices

The process of urbanisation made them to adapt the modern methods of treatment wherever the modern medical facility have been provided. However, before the process of urbanisation the Banjaras have depended totally on the indigenous methods of cure such as magico-religious and herbal medicines. Even child birth were assisted by the local midwives; whose main qualifications were advanced age and experience of having given birth to more number of children. Banjaras say that if any misfortune was interpreted its because of an act of evil spirit or due to fate. The settlement as a whole acts as one ritual unit and the Banjaras totally depend on the deity of the settlement for the protection and welfare of individual's commitment.

The rituals and festivals in these settlements are either curative or preventive. Every year the festival of the village deity is celebrated on a grand scale and large number of animals and food items are offered to please the deity. It is believed that the troubles such as diseases to man and animals, failures of rains and crops are caused by the evil spirits and displeased ancestors. Normally the evil beings resided outside the ritual boundary of the settlements and settlement deity was vested with the responsibility of keeping them away. When displeased with man's behaviour or morals, the deity abstained from performing her roles and thus permitted the entry of evil spirits into the settlement.

For health problems of magic-religious nature, they take the help of shaman and priests. For other problems they go for herbal medicine. With their knowledge for the locally available herbs and minerals, Banjaras use them as cure for their discomforts. Traditional medical practitioners were experienced and aged and had learnt the art of treating the patients from their forefathers. The cure was provided as a moral obligation towards their fellow residents and did not expect anything in return.

The process of urbanisation made Banjaras in the settlement to concentrate more on personal and community hygiene as well as nutrition. They go to the adjacent towns and hospitals for acquiring many new concepts of planned settlement and education in health and hygiene. In the beginning, hospitals were functioning only in the district and taluk, but now planning to introduce health administration at different levels from village panchayat up to state levels. However, traditional aged Banjaras were slow in accepting the new methods since this system of medicine and cure was different from their own. The process of urbanisation not only made them to accept the western method of cure but also started paying for that in the form of cess, tax and fee to the state.

In accordance with the development programmes of the welfare state which was adopted after the independence of India, many health programmes were started. Among them establishment of the health department and directorates, nursing schools, medical colleges and maintaining budget provision for health and separate ministry as well as issuing of licenses to pharmaceutical laboratories, etc. Mass immunisation and health education programmes were also taken up under aid from WHO. Extension of health facilities to rural areas by creating primary health units for every one lakh of population at villages and starting of medical dispensaries for every 10,000 population was another step forward. As of now there are 236 hospitals, 1,554 primary health units and 364 primary health centres in the State today (Government of Karnataka, 1985). But so far no single health unit is found in the settlements of Banjaras.

Medical dispensary was opened at villages, near by Banjara settlements of Bellary District in Karnataka. Since there was no building readily available to house it, the village panchayat office building was vacated and was made available for the dispensary. Another building which was being used earlier as a school house, was also vacated and made available for the doctor's residence. This caused lot of problems to the panchayat and school authorities and even resulted in factional feuds at village level, due to which, Banjaras stopped visiting the medical dispensaries. As a result of all these problems, though it got a medical dispensary and the services of a qualified doctor for the benefit of the people, no doctor who was posted to the village lived here. Rather they preferred to commute daily from the towns. Further they also took transfer out of villages, to a better place or town on the plea that the village has no good school for their children, no good transportation facility and so on. So far eight doctors were posted to villages, near Banjara settlements and among them only one doctor opted to stay with his family in the village. During the absence of the doctor, the midwife and the compounder in the dispensary play the role of a doctor and provides the medical aid to the patients which was improper and also sometimes might prove dangerous. The officials and the village leaders overlooked this aspect as they thought some medical aid was available even in the absence of the doctor in the village.

Owing to uncertainty of the availability of the doctors as well as medicine in the village dispensary, the patients from village, from Banjara settlements and from neighbouring villages attached to the dispensary, go to the respective taluka by buses and bullock carts to obtain medical aid. They were directed to hospitals and specialists in the town whenever patients were serious or no medicines were available locally. It is the opinion of Banjaras that at district hospitals the facilities like wards, x-ray and surgical facilities were available. These facilities were not provided at village dispensary and the doctors who worked here were not specialists. Though it was a wrong policy to concentrate all the medical facilities in one place, that too in towns, the government went ahead opening large number of hospitals in urban centres. As a result the patients from rural areas undergo lot of trouble to avail these facilities today.

Acceptance of western method of clinical cure has adversely affected the economy of Banjaras of Karnataka. To get good care and facilities the patients are asked to go to hospitals and specialists in urban centres. The specialists in turn ask the patients to get themselves admitted to wards for proper investigation. In some cases the patients are asked to stay in the hospitals for days and weeks to get the continuous medical or surgical treatment. In order to look after the patient one or two of his relatives also stay with him in the hospital. This poses certain problems, such as sharing of the limited space and facilities and botheration to the patient. Moreover it increases lot of expenditure on the patient's family and often they are led either to borrow heavily or part with gold or landed property. Staying of more number of able bodied members away from home and farm work also amounts to financial loss to the family. Banjaras of Karnataka say that when they stay in urban hospital wards, it poses many difficulties. Being orthodox they often refuse to accept food and milk which are freely provided in public hospitals. Lack of communication skills to contact the hospital staff and administrators to make use of the ward and other facilities also results in problems to them. Even the visiting hours fixed by the urban hospital are not convenient to them since they have to take buses and trains which are not under their control to reach here on time. So they often return home without seeing their sick relatives. This failure means violation of kin and community obligations. A patient usually expects that his close clan members is to visit him and give moral support during his hour of trouble and sometimes, last days. When they fail to do so it brings conflicts in their relations. To overcome all these problems the Banjaras prefer private nursing homes, where the restrictions are not strictly maintained by the hospital staff. But availing the facilities in private nursing homes means heavy expenditure.

Diet and nourishment are closely related to modern clinical cure. Doctors prescribe vitamins, tonic and nutritious foods without realising the socio-economic conditions of the patients. They also fail to understand that these requirements can be met by consuming locally available fruits, vegetables and home-made food items which could be obtained not only cheaply but also in fresh condition.

Establishment of big urban hospitals has also given rise to many human problems. Location of latest and specialised medical facilities attracts large number of patients from far and near. Lack of human consideration among the medical staff in these hospitals is the main cause of many problems (c.f., Desai, 1988). The staff fails to realise that the patients in a ward is from a closely knit social group. A patient from rural background, who is used to personal and continuous attention from the indigenous curers, begins to feel that he is being neglected by the doctors who visit the patients once or at the most twice a day and for the rest of the whole day the patients are left in the care of the nursing and technical staff (Gurumurthy, 1976). Often the huge building and staff baffle them. A patient feels helpless when he is tossed from one counter to another to fill forms, pay bills and to consult specialists.

There are other problems also brought by larger hospitals. When electricity fails, x-ray and other equipments break down; the entire technical equipment gets paralysed. Technicians to repair them have to be called from far-off cities. The management also takes its own time to give administrative sanction to get these machines repaired. The staff of the hospitals often goes on strike on minor issues and hampers the working of the hospitals. Admission of large number of patients in the hospital makes it impossible for the specialists to give individual attention to each patient. Often patients in big hospitals, and especially in the teaching hospitals, are left to the care of the junior doctors and students. If the hygienic condition in the hospitals is not maintained well, infection which sets in one ward or operation theatre is likely to spread to others. These have been highlighted by certain commissions instituted by a few state governments. In a country like India, where the people still believe in fate and where health insurance has not become popular, the poor and ignorant patients suffer in terms of health and monetary loss. All these make the patients and their kin to adopt a negative attitude towards the modern clinical cure.

Presence of big hospitals in towns and cities, which are also business and industrial centres, presents problems to the citizens of these urban areas. To avail medical, surgical, maternity and dental treatment, thousands of patients visit the town everyday. During their stay the city dwellers are faced with a number of hardships since they have to share the already limited civic amenities available with the local residents. Thus the medical system has brought in its way a chain of problems for the management of which anthropological skills and insights hold a great promise.

Summary and Conclusion

Traditional societies tend to be well adapted to those aspects of their immediate environments that are relevant to health and survival. They continually interact with and adjust by cultural and biological means to the existing populations of microorganisms and vectors and to the life-supporting fauna and flora. 'Adaptation' here means coexistence with these populations, maintenance of ecological complexity, and resource management. The good health of the members of traditional societies is, however, not a state characterised by the absence of disease but a state of benign chronic and endemic. It is not a state of extermination of disease but one of steady control at bearable levels. Urbanising societies lose this type of adaptation. Their cultural and biological repertoires are no longer capable of dealing with sudden environmental alterations or cultural intrusions originating from powerful outside sources. New populations of microorganisms are introduced. Organisms already present may find the changed conditions more favourable for their breeding and/or transmission, and the same may hold for vector populations. Epidemics are therefore an early risk. In addition, man made environmental changes usually reduce ecological complexity, and a fauna and flora thus impoverished may constitute the risk of malnutrition. Many cultural changes have been detrimental to health and nutrition. Among these are the adoption of a sedentary lifestyle, the growing preference for imported carbohydrate staples, and the increasing use of infant formulas, the reluctance to breastfeed for long periods, the abolition of native family planning methods, the acceptance of paid work, and the eagerness to grow cash crops.

Urbanising societies either perish or find ways to adapt to their new environment. But since their effective environment now encompasses the whole world, with all its unpredictable turmoil and uncontrollable changes, they may never again achieve a balanced state of adaptation.

It is ironic that for a long time anthropologists regarded un-urbanised traditional hunter-gatherer societies (and, for that matter, traditional horticulturalists) as 'evolutionary failures eking out an impoverished existence in the more remote and marginal regions of the world' (Tonkinson, 1983). Only recently have anthropologists begun to recognise their success. They attribute the health and vigour of such people and their lack of major nutritional deficiencies and modern ailments mostly to such cultural adaptations as geographic isolation, small group size, nomadic lifestyle, diverse diet, and a preservative attitude towards the environment. They also recognise the presence of biological adaptations to certain infections and nutritional shortcomings.

Un-urbanised traditional societies are not free of disease. They suffer infection by an impressive array of infectious agents and minor nutritional deficiencies. However, they have found a way to coexist with their microorganisms and to live with their nutritional shortcomings without much visible morbidity and death. Since such societies have long been in constant interaction with their immediate environments, it can be assumed that the majority of their diseases will evolve either towards extinction or more likely towards becoming less pathological and virulent. In a modern, less adapted civilised population, infection with the same gamut of microbial agents would probably take a much heavier toll in morbidity and death (Neel and Salzano, 1967).

In the olden days unacculturated traditional societies like Banjaras managed their health care through indigenous systems conducted by the native priests, shamans and herbalarious. The care and treatment were easily and locally available with minimum cost. Their concepts of prevention of diseases and maintenance of cleanliness are closely linked to the other aspects of their social life. The food habits were in accordance with the local customs and values. Since the cure was offered nearer to home there was no necessity of spending on the stay in hospitals and also on transportation of the patient and his kin from one place to another. However, of urbanised clinical cure, which is a part of total westernisation process, the people in the traditional way of life are put to quite a few hardships. First, they are at a loss to perceive the aspects of health, hygiene and nutrition which are not related in their worldview and are being recognised as scientifically separate. They are neither educated about the urbanised system nor provided with the required facilities to fully utilise the modern clinical cure. Secondly they have to bear huge costs on western medicine and hospital facilities. Further, they are made to go to towns and cities to get the cure from hospitals which in its process create many socio-cultural problems.

By totally accepting and supporting the western medicare system, the governments of Third World countries have unintentionally created many problems in health care and management. Without a proper understanding of their local problems and a valid estimation of their present needs in respect of clinical cure, the governments established large hospitals in towns and cities where industries, trade and commerce agencies are also located. The location of larger hospitals in towns with many specialists, wards, x-ray and surgical facilities was effected without keeping in mind the efficiency, fuller use of the facility and their economy. For most of the Third World societies, all these facilities could certainly be made suitable with certain adjustments keeping in view their socio-cultural conditions. To bring the patients, one or two kinsmen invariably accompany him for which huge amount of money has to be paid in the form of fee and charges on medicines. Communication with hospital staff and stay in the wards with many sick and terminal patients is few other problems that people need to face.

Often administration and management of larger hospitals in most of the Third World countries becomes problematic because of their own but 'unsuitable' economic systems, problems of inadequate electricity, illiteracy, lack of education in advanced science and technology, lack of general awareness about health and hygiene, exorbitant hospital charges in terms of currency as well as peculiarities of native disease cycles. In many cases these difficulties have promoted the general public to form a negative opinion about the hospitals and the urban curative systems. Nevertheless they are left with no alternative but to continue to accept this method of cure since the indigenous methods have gradually been lost or are being disbelieved. The urban clinical cure as a part of westernisation process seems to have come to stay. This has more often than not resulted in the exploitation of rural patients. To avoid the use of costly and strong drugs and their side effects, some even settle with the services of quacks. Therefore, a proper understanding of socio-cultural factors as well as an adequate assessment of the felt needs and capacities of the people who accept the western medical system is necessary to manage it usefully and meaningfully.

References

Desai, Anita. 1988. Big Hospitals: For Whose Benefit. *Indian Express*, 6 June , p. 8.

Gurumurthy, K.G. 1976. *Kallapura: A South Indian Village*. Karnatak University Press, Dharwad.

Government of Karnataka. 1985. *Karnataka at a Glance, 1984–85*. Directorate of Economics and Statistics, Bangalore.

Jagadeesh, V. 2005. *The Study of Lamani Tribe: An Anthropological Perspective*. Sona Book House, Bangalore.

Neel, J.V. and F.M. Salzano. 1967. Further Studies on the Xavante Indians. X. Some Hypotheses-generalizations Resulting from these Studies. *American Journal of Human Genetics*, 19: 554–74.

Tonkinson, R. 1983. Hunter-gatherers in Modern Settings (Book review of *Politics and History in Band Societies*, edited by E. Leacock and R. Lee) *Science*, 220 (4602): 1143–44.

Index